Lecture Notes in Bioinformatics 8574

Subseries of Lecture Notes in Computer Science

Helena Galhardas   Erhard Rahm (Eds.)

Data Integration in the Life Sciences

10th International Conference, DILS 2014
Lisbon, Portugal, July 17-18, 2014
Proceedings

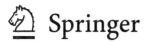 Springer

Volume Editors

Helena Galhardas
Instituto Superior Técnico, University of Lisbon
INESC-ID
Tagus Park
Av. Prof. Dr. Cavaco Silva
2744-016 Porto Salvo, Portugal
E-mail: helena.galhardas@tecnico.ulisboa.pt

Erhard Rahm
Universität Leipzig
Fakultät für Mathematik und Informatik
Institut für Informatik
Augustusplatz 10
04109 Leipzig, Germany
E-mail: rahm@informatik.uni-leipzig.de

ISSN 0302-9743   e-ISSN 1611-3349
ISBN 978-3-319-08589-0   e-ISBN 978-3-319-08590-6
DOI 10.1007/978-3-319-08590-6
Springer Cham Heidelberg New York Dordrecht London

Library of Congress Control Number: 2014941868

LNCS Sublibrary: SL 8 – Bioinformatics

Typesetting: Camera-ready by author, data conversion by Scientific Publishing Services, Chennai, India

Printed on acid-free paper

Springer is part of Springer Science+Business Media (www.springer.com)

Preface

This volume of *Lecture Notes in Bioinformatics* (LNBI) contains the papers presented at DILS 2014: the 10th International Conference on Data Integration in the Life Sciences, held during July 16–17, 2014 in Lisbon, Portugal. In its 10th year, DILS was hosted at Instituto Superior Técnico, University of Lisbon (http://dils2014.inesc-id.pt) and chaired by Erhard Rahm and Helena Galhardas.

The first edition of DILS took place in 2004 in Leipzig, Germany. Over the years, the conference continued to foster discussion, exchange, and innovation in research and development in the areas of data integration and data management in the life sciences. These topics have become more and more important due to the increasing availability of Big Data, coming from high-throughput analytical techniques, large clinical data repositories, biomedical literature and online resources, that offer exciting opportunities and challenges to researchers and professionals from biology, medicine, computer science, and engineering. So far the conference took place in five European countries (Germany, UK, France, Sweden, Portugal), in the USA (three times) and in Canada making DILS a truly international forum.

This year, DILS was a forum that put together invited keynote presentations, oral presentations of peer-reviewed research, application and systems papers, poster and demo presentations. Each submission was reviewed by three Program Committee members. After a careful evaluation process, the Program Committee decided to accept 14 long and short papers that are included in this volume. The accepted papers cover interesting and current topics: data integration platforms and applications, biodiversity data management methods and applications, biomedical ontologies, linked data integration, visualization techniques, and scientific data retrieval and querying. DILS 2014 also included several poster and demo contributions on work-in-progress and system prototypes. The accepted poster and demo papers are published on the conference website.

DILS 2014 featured two distinguished keynote speakers: Dr. Alfonso Valencia and Prof. Jonas S. Almeida. Dr. Alfonso Valencia, vice-director of Basic Research and director of the Structural Biology and Biocomputing Program of the Spanish National Cancer Research Center (CNIO), is an expert in applying computational methods and tools to the analysis of large collections of genomic information, in particular to study protein families and protein interaction networks. His recent research focus is in the domain of cancer (epi)genomics, tumor evolution and precision medicine. In his talk, Dr. Valencia presented the challenges and opportunities of Computational Biology and Big Data. Specifically, he pointed out how technology has influenced the development of Biomedicine and Ecology areas and the current limitations for dealing with large, complex, heterogeneous and low quality data sets and the urge for additional knowledge to interpret the results obtained. Prof. Jonas S. Almeida, Director of the division in Informatics of the Department of Pathology of the University of Alabama at Birmingham (UAB), is specialized on integrative personalized medicine applications. Prof. Almeida has a strong background on all components of quantitative Biology ranging from experimentation, engineering and mathematical modeling to computational statistics and software engineering. His current research interests are on the synergy obtained by combining Semantic Web abstractions and Distributed Cloud Computing approaches to Bioinformatics applications. In his talk, Prof. Almeida overviewed recent solutions in Biomedicine with a particular emphasis on Semantic Web frameworks and code distribution.

As the event co-chairs and editors of this volume, we would like to thank all authors who submitted papers, as well as the Program Committee members and additional referees for their excellent contribution in evaluating the submissions. Special thanks go to INESC-ID and Instituto Superior Técnico, University of Lisbon for providing us with the facilities to organize and run the event. We would also like to thank FCT (*Fundação para a Ciência e Tecnologia*) for the financial support provided, in particular through the excellence research network "DataStorm - Large-Scale Data Management in Cloud Environments". We would also like to thank Alfred Hofmann and his team at Springer for their continued cooperation and help in putting this volume together. We also thank the Easy-Chair team for having developed this tool that enabled us to smoothly manage submissions, reviews and proceedings. Finally, our thanks go to the local Organizing Committee, Ana Teresa Freitas, José Borbinha, José Leal, Mário J. Silva and Pedro T. Monteiro, our Webmaster, João L.M. Pereira, and our administrative staff from INESC-ID, Manuela Sado and Sandra Sá.

July 2014   Helena Galhardas
                                                                              Erhard Rahm

Organization

Program Committee Chair

Helena Galhardas | INESC-ID and Instituto Superior Técnico,
University of Lisbon, Portugal
Erhard Rahm | University of Leipzig, Germany

Program Committee

Christopher Baker | University of New Brunswick, Canada
Kenneth J. Barker | IBM, USA
Olivier Bodenreider | NIH, USA
João Carriço | IMM, Portugal
Claudine Chaouiya | IGC, Portugal
James Cimino | National Library of Medicine, USA
Luis Pedro Coelho | EMBL, Germany
Sarah Cohen-Boulakia | LRI, University of Paris-Sud 11, France
Francisco Couto | Faculty of Sciences, University of Lisbon, Portugal
Alexandre Francisco | INESC-ID and Instituto Superior Técnico, University of Lisbon, Portugal
Juliana Freire | NYU-Poly, USA
Christine Froidevaux | LRI University of Paris-Sud 11, France
Hasan Jamil | University of Idaho, USA
Graham Kemp | Chalmers University of Technology, Sweden
Toralf Kirsten | University of Leipzig, Germany
Birgitta König-Ries | Friedrich-Schiller-Universität Jena, Germany
Patrick Lambrix | Linköping University, Sweden
Adam Lee | University of Maryland and National Library of Medicine, USA
Mong Li Lee | National University of Singapore, Singapore
Ulf Leser | Humboldt University, Germany
Bertram Ludaescher | University of California, USA
Paolo Missier | Newcastle University, UK
Norman Paton | University of Manchester, UK
Cédric Prusky | CRP Henri Tudor, Luxemburg
Uwe Scholz | IPK Gatersleben, Germany
Maria Esther Vidal | Universidad Simón Bolívar, Venezuela
Dagmar Waltemath | University of Rostock, Germany

Additional Reviewers

Daniel Faria	Faculty of Sciences, University of Lisbon, Portugal
David Koop	NYU-Poly, USA
Catia Pesquita	Faculty of Sciences, University of Lisbon, Portugal
Emanuel Santos	Faculty of Sciences, University of Lisbon, Portugal
Martin Scharm	University of Rostock, Germany
Cátia Vaz	ISEL, Polytechnic Institute of Lisbon, Portugal

DILS Steering Committee

Christopher Baker	University of New Brunswick, Canada
Sarah Cohen-Boulakia	LRI, University of Paris-Sud 11, France
Graham Kemp	Chalmers University of Technology, Sweden
Ulf Leser	Humboldt University, Germany
Paolo Missier	Newcastle University, UK
Norman Paton	University of Manchester, UK
Erhard Rahm	University of Leipzig, Germany
Louiqa Raschid	University of Maryland, USA

Organizing Committee

José Borbinha	INESC-ID and Instituto Superior Técnico, University of Lisbon, Portugal
Ana Teresa Freitas	INESC-ID and Instituto Superior Técnico, University of Lisbon, Portugal
José Leal	Instituto Gulbenkian de Ciência, Portugal
Pedro T. Monteiro	INESC-ID, Portugal
Mário J. Silva	INESC-ID and Instituto Superior Técnico, University of Lisbon, Portugal

Webmaster

João L.M. Pereira	INESC-ID and Instituto Superior Técnico, University of Lisbon, Portugal

Keynote Papers

Computational Biology and Big Data: Challenges and Opportunities

Alfonso Valencia

Spanish National Cancer Research Center
valencia@cnio.es

Abstract. Technology is influencing the development of all areas from Biomedicine to Ecology and transforming Biology in a quantitative science. This accelerated technical progression is reflected in the rapid succession of keywords that went in the 20 years from "genomics" to "proteomics", "systems biology" and "synthetic biology" to the current "big data". All of them paving the way to deciphering the function biological systems, from cells to ecosystems, based on the integration of data on genomes, proteomes, metabolomes, environments and conditions.

A promising future that is limited by: a) the current computational technologies for handling large, complex and heterogeneous and in many cases low quality data, and b) very important, the insufficiency of the biological knowledge necessary to interpret the results. In this scenario Bioinformatics and Computational Biology play a central rôle. A particularly good example is the complex task of individual genomes analysis, which involves data organization, integration and interpretation. A challenge that touches many areas of computation and informatics and requires a blend of engineering and scientific developments.

Genome projects are a good example of projects that deal with large scale data, that can be considered part of the Big Data movement. Based on the experience of my group in these projects I will review both the technical framework for handling genomic information and the methods required for the interpretation of the information. In particular, I will focus discuss some of the key scientific problems in the analysis of high-throughput genotype-phenotype information oriented to the prediction of genomics basis of disease conditions.

References

1. Valencia, A., Hidalgo, M.: Getting personalized cancer genome analysis into the clinic: the challenges in Bioinformatics. Genome Medicine, 461 (2012)
2. Vazquez, M., de la Torre, V., Valencia, A.: Cancer Genome Analysis. In: Translational Bioinformatics PLOS Computational Biology Open Access Book, ch. 14 (2012)
3. de Juan, D., Pazos, F., Valencia, A.: Emerging methods in protein co-evolution. Nat. Rev. Genet. 14, 249–261 (2013)
4. Rodriguez, J.M., Maietta, P., Ezkurdia, I., Pietrelli, A., Wesselink, J.J., Lopez, G., Valencia, A., Tress, M.L.: APPRIS: annotation of principal and alternative splice isoforms. Nucleic Acids Res. 41, D110–D117 (2013)

5. Ibañez, C., Boullosa, C., Tabarés-Seisdedos, R., Baudot, A., Valencia, A.: Molecular Evidence for the Inverse Comorbidity between Central Nervous System Disorders and Cancers detected by Transcriptomic Meta-analyses. Plos Genet. 10, e1004173 (2014)

The Emergence of the Web Computer: An Hands-on View from the Trenches of Computational Pathology

Jonas S. Almeida

Div. Informatics, Dept. Pathology, Univ. Birmingham at Birmingham
`jalmeida@uab.edu`

Abstract. The need to contextualize data about an experiment or a patient is increasingly achieved with reference to Big Data resources such as The Cancer Genome Atlas (TCGA). This exercise faces numerous obstacles, from the logistics of traversing a very large and constantly growing data set (the number of files hosted by TCGA doubles every 7 months [1]) to the protection of patient privacy. It also includes an absolute need for "weak AI" to reach domain experts increasingly immersed in mobile platforms. These challenges are not unique to Biomedicine but are, in many regards, particularly difficult to meet in this domain [2]. Correspondingly, the pursuit of solutions is part of the core mission of the new sub-discipline of Computational Pathology [3]. This presentation will overview early stage solutions with applications ranging from image analysis in cytology [4] and sequence analysis [5] to the personalization of cancer treatment. These illustrative applications will be used as part of an argument for the central role played by Web Technologies, with particular emphasis on Semantic Web frameworks and code distribution directly to the ubiquitous Web Platform supported by the modern web browser.

References

1. Robbins, D.E., Grüneberg, A., Deus, H.F., Tanik, M.M., Almeida, J.S.: A self-updating road map of The Cancer Genome Atlas. Bioinformatics 29(10), 1333–1340 (2013)
2. Almeida, J.S., Dress, A., Kühne, T., Parida, L.: ICT for Bridging Biology and Medicine. Dagstuhl Manifestos 3(1), 31–50 (2014)
3. Park, S., Parwani, A.V., Aller, R.D., Banach, L., Becich, M.J., Borkenfeld, S., et al.: The history of pathology informatics: A global perspective. Journal of Pathology Informatics 4 (2013)
4. Almeida, J.S., Iriabho, E.E., Gorrepati, V.L., Wilkinson, S.R., Grüneberg, A., Robbins, D.E., et al.: ImageJS: personalized, participated, pervasive, and reproducible image bioinformatics in the web browser. Journal of Pathology Informatics 3 (2012)
5. Almeida, J.S., Grüneberg, A., Maass, W., Vinga, S.: Fractal MapReduce decomposition of sequence alignment. Algorithms for Molecular Biology 7, 12 (2012)

Table of Contents

Linked Data and Query Processing

An Asset Management Approach to Continuous Integration of Heterogeneous Biomedical Data

Robert E. Schuler, Carl Kesselman, and Karl Czajkowski

Information Sciences Institute, University of Southern California
{schuler,carl,karlcz}@isi.edu

Abstract. Increasingly, advances in biomedical research are the result of combining and analyzing heterogeneous data types from different sources, spanning genomic, proteomic, imaging, and clinical data. Yet despite the proliferation of data-driven methods, tools to support the integration and management of large collections of data for purposes of data driven discovery are scarce, leaving scientists with ad hoc and inefficient processes. The scientific process could benefit significantly from lightweight methods for data integration that allow for exploratory, incrementally refined integration of heterogeneous data. In this paper, we address this problem by introducing a new asset management based approach designed to support continuous integration of biomedical data. We describe the system and our experiences using it in the context of several scientific applications.

1   Introduction

Biomedical advances are driven at the intersections of data: combining imaging, genetic, clinical, and other sources in cross cutting analytic methods. It is not uncommon to see a dozen different types of biomedical data, spanning genetics, multiple imaging modalities, proteomics, and clinical elements, being used in a single exploration or discovery process, each data with its own unique representation. A logical prerequisite for analysis is that the necessary data has been integrated into a formal, standard, clean, consistent, accessible, and linked representation prior to analysis. However, the vast majority of scientific data in daily use does not exist in a manner that meets even a few, if any, of the above characteristics. It is widely understood that "data wrangling" is often the most resource intensive activity in data analysis – a time-consuming process of data selection, transformation, and cleansing. All too often it is only at the very end of the scientific discovery process, while preparing data for submission into online repositories that data is integrated, organized, and annotated according to overarching standard dictionaries, ontologies, and open formats. Instead throughout most of the scientific processes, the vast majority of research data exist in semistructured, locally coded sources and formats. One consequence is that scientists often spend significant amounts of their research time managing, combining, and manipulating data, with self-reported values of 90% being common [1]. With the increasing proliferation of large biomedical data (e.g. big data), the problems will only grow worse.

H. Galhardas and E. Rahm (Eds.): DILS 2014, LNBI 8574, pp. 1–15, 2014.

In spite of this situation, it is remarkable that there is little support for scientists to integrate and organize data for purposes of exploration, analysis, and ultimate publication. Shared file systems with data organized in directory hierarchies and with metadata coded into "meaningful" file names are the common practice. Idiosyncratic methods are used to capture and unify pertinent metadata such as phenotype, experiment details, preparation methods, and quality control flags. All too often spreadsheets, which are hard to maintain and offer limited query ability, are the preferred means of describing and tracking data. Cloud based services such as Dropbox and Google Drive can provide some relief with respect to sharing, but do little to address the fundamental issues of integration and organization.

This paper presents a system that fills this gap by enabling continuous integration of heterogeneous biomedical data throughout the research and discovery lifecycle. This "pay-as-you-go" approach, influenced by the concept of Dataspaces [2], uses a process of incremental refinement to promote flexible, use-case driven data integration, which can mesh with the requirements of the data task at hand. To maximize the use of these methods by scientists, we have incorporated them into a digital asset management system for biomedical data (BDAM) that resembles cloud based tools and services with which investigators are already familiar. The structure of this paper is as follows. In Section 2, we introduce the concept of digital asset management and continuous integration to build a unified view over heterogeneous life science data collections. In Section 3, we discuss related work. Section 4, presents design of a biomedical digital asset management system whose application in a range of use cases is discussed in Section 5. Finally we describe future plans and conclusions .

2   Asset Management Method for Continuous Integration

Digital asset management (DAM) "consists of management tasks and decisions surrounding the ingestion, annotation, cataloguing, storage, retrieval and distribution of digital assets" [3]. DAM systems are designed to streamline free-form "creative" processes rather than enforce predefined business processes. DAM is nearly ubiquitous for many varieties and applications of data, from text and document management to multimedia to specialized systems for marketing and the web. For example, DAM systems for photo management like iPhoto or Picasa will discover and catalog digital images on one's hard disk drive, extract metadata from the imported media, cleanse (fix or add missing) metadata, allow user annotations (typically in the form of tags), organize pictures into virtual collections (i.e. photo albums), support browsing and search, support data export for data manipulation by external photo editing tools, and support publication for cloud based sharing or printing by online services.

Surprisingly, in spite of the fact that there would seem to be a good alignment between the data management requirements for biomedical discovery and the functions provided by DAM systems, DAM approaches have not been generally applied to biomedical data management. Building on the success of DAM in other creative fields, we claim that an approach to data integration that assists scientists throughout the research lifecycle based on a biomedical digital asset management system (BDAM) would significantly streamline the process of data driven scientific discovery in the life sciences. However, it is also the case that simply applying an existing

DAM technology will be insufficient to meet the needs of life sciences where the data are both large and significantly more diverse.

2.1 Continuous Integration of Biomedical Data

As discussed above, a core requirement of BDAM is the ability to manage a heterogeneous collection of asset types, each with their own characteristics, descriptive metadata, and storage representation (i.e. file format). Within the overall function of asset management, one can take a broad perspective of what it means to provide integration based on the management operations under consideration: i.e. search, organization, or export for analysis. We may limit integration to the descriptive metadata associated with each asset (or collection of assets) or we may want to provide a uniform rendering of the structure of the asset itself. For example, assets of diverse types can be integrated simply by being grouped into logical collections, assets may be collected based on shared common attributes and criteria (i.e. faceted search [4]), or the underlying structure of the assets themselves may be transformed, transcoded, or reformatted into a uniform representation.

Common approaches to data integration, which depend on tight semantic integration of traditional database Extraction-Transformation-Loading (ETL), upfront semantic alignment and schema mapping (e.g., query mediation [5]) are problematic when the descriptive data is not known beforehand, or may change during the discovery process, which is often the case in life sciences application. Consequently, an incremental model which assumes that metadata is incomplete [6] or evolving [7], that assumes loose semantic integration, no upfront semantic alignment, loose administrative proximity, and loose consistency with sources will have broader applicability than a non-incremental approach. Building on the axiom of "integrate early and often" approaches such as Dataspaces [2] or MAD [8] seek to accelerate the use of data by deferring integration until required. We embrace this model as a core aspect of BDAM by providing functions for editing, augmenting, and refining metadata descriptions incrementally over the lifetime of the discovery process. This is not to say that established models cannot be used, even in early phases of data use. With BDAM we take a hybrid approach where structured metadata is ingested into the system and augmented with incrementally defined descriptions.

3   Related Work

Digital repository systems (e.g. DSpace [9]) provide capabilities aimed at long-term preservation and archiving of scholarly works. They are primarily concerned with document management (Word, PDF, JPEG, etc.), whereas a DAM system for life sciences must support diverse biomedical file formats and very large file sizes and overall file volumes. Digital repositories support publication and archiving, thus they should be viewed as an endpoint for the scientific data assets produced by researchers. Plale et al [7] have proposed the SEAD Virtual Archive for federating institutional repositories along with automated workflows to assist researchers in the data publication process. The asset management approach proposed here takes this a significant step further by pushing deeper and earlier into the scientific discovery process so that data curation is not an overhead but an integral part of the discovery processes.

SQLShare [1] is a system that has many elements in common with the BDAM catalog including the concepts of schema evolution and incremental refinement. However, SQLShare differs from our work in several significant ways. It focuses on SQL as the primary interface by which users interact and assumes that the data of interest is primarily stored in the SQLShare database. Metadata catalogs, such as Globus Metadata Catalog Service were proposed [10], with an extensible schema as a general purpose tool to support data management in e-sciences. The asset management approach argues that metadata catalogs must be coupled with semi-automated methods for metadata ingest and complementary asset management services.

Picture Archiving and Communications Systems (PACS) based on the DICOM standard for medical imaging interoperability offer clinical image management services with interfaces to store, query, and retrieve radiology images. Related are research systems such as XNAT [11]. These systems, however, are focused almost exclusively on radiology imaging rather than other imaging modalities or data types, and they do not offer schema evolution, as described later.

Finally, storage management systems, including SRM [12], and iRODS [13], provide facilities for lower-level data storage operations and storage resource management. They generally operate on data at a semantically lower level than digital asset management and offer limited facilities for metadata management.

4   BDAM Design and Implementation

The core elements of any DAM system include: 1) a catalog for tracking, managing and organizing assets, 2) ingest methods for incorporating data assets into the system

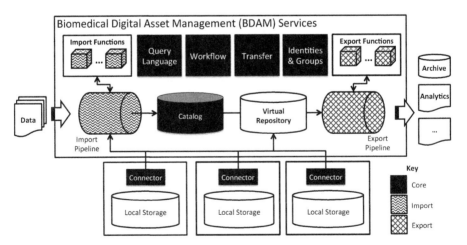

Fig. 1. The architecture of a biomedical digital asset management service. BDAM services are loosely coupled via connectors to local storage and they facilitate import and export pipelines with extensible functions.

and extracting basic descriptive metadata, 3) storage services for storing and moving assets, and 4) methods for extracting assets from the system for analysis and publication. Pervasive across all these functions must be methods for specifying and enforcing policy for access and use. The relationship between these functions is shown in Fig 1.

4.1 Design Requirements

The heterogeneity of data assets and scientific processes means that the semantic and syntactic models for metadata and data are often not known a priori. Furthermore, the metadata characterizing a particular asset and its relationship to the research or discovery task at hand is not a simple functional product of the data content but may vary depending on the research questions being posed and the kind of data discovery that will be performed. We adopt a *relaxed consistency* model in which a data asset continually evolves, rather than entering the system fully formed and with all metadata predetermined. We allow *incremental refinement* of content and schema, throughout scientific discovery.

The disparate sources of data assets are not always under one administrative domain. Scientific discovery may involve assets located in a combination of local, enterprise and cloud based storage. In many cases restricted access data covered by Institutional Review Boards, government regulations such as Health Insurance Portability and Accountability Act, and other Data Use Agreements may not permit the use of clouds for storage of sensitive data. We adopt a hybrid design [14] with *loose coupling*, in which core components are operated in a software-as-a-service (SaaS) platform while user data may reside in local storage services (see Fig. 1). The complexities of managing the core services are reduced by operating in a hosted environment, while institutional data access controls are preserved and storage costs are lowered.

In addition to schema evolution, the BDAM must support *schema introspection*. Given the dynamic nature of schema evolution, the applications and user interfaces must be able to inspect the catalog's schema and present interfaces for the user to query and manipulate content. Often, useful metadata that characterizes data assets may contain private information, and it is not enough to assume access control for data assets while having unrestricted access to metadata. A BDAM must support *fine-grain access control* to restrict access to metadata about specific assets (e.g. rows or resources), to attributes (e.g. columns or property types) of the any asset, or to whole collection of metadata (e.g. tables or graphs). Data storage services should support complementary access control to the data.

Finally, if a BDAM is offered as a shared service it must support *multi-tenancy* to allow each scientific application to operate at its own pace and with its own content and access policies. All these design characteristics (loose coupling, relaxed consistency, incremental refinement, fine-grain access control, and multi-tenancy) complement one another. The BDAM is able to capture the evolving state of the scientific discovery process as data assets are acquired, summarized, queried, processed, and analyzed by researchers.

4.2   Data Catalog

The BDAM data catalog allows individual data assets or other relevant resources to be recorded along with meaningful metadata descriptions. As one of the loosely coupled components of the BDAM, the catalog may receive input from multiple sources including direct, user-authored metadata and machine-driven metadata extraction tools. These catalog contents can be browsed or searched to find assets matching certain criteria. The catalog schema can be queried and amended as per our schema evolution and introspection design requirements. Metadata concepts must be defined before first use, but these definitions can be incrementally added to the running catalog at any point during its operation.

In keeping with the SaaS model, interactions with the catalog are via a RESTful web services protocol. The catalog contains metadata records as resources which can be manipulated by the client. The defined interface includes functions for retrieving and amending the metadata schema; creating, destroying, updating, and retrieving whole metadata records; updating or retrieving individual metadata properties for specific records; or performing queries of the records by metadata criteria and associations to other contextual records. The metadata update and retrieval interfaces also allow bulk operations to efficiently manipulate many records in a single request.

We have developed and evaluated two distinct catalog implementations, both presenting a web service access protocol on top of a relational database management system (RDBMS). Based on the widespread appeal of graph-base query in data integration, we initially explored sparse data storage models with a graph-based query interface, which we called Tagfiler (described later). However, we found that in practice, many investigations use a handful of dominant resource models where many assets were annotated with the same subset of metadata concepts. In such an environment, it is desirable to use a more compact representation of metadata. Consequently, we developed an alternative catalog interface which supports more structured modeling of data. *ERMrest*, a portmanteau of ERM (Entity Relationship Model) and REST (REpresentational State Transfer) exposes a table-like concept of typed entities with type-specific properties and is tuned for dense metadata by storing entities and their properties as rows in conventional tables.

In both ERMrest and Tagfiler, the catalog model exposes not only individually named metadata records, but also complex record sets. Both also support complex query patterns where assets can be found not only by their direct metadata but also by their relationships to other matching assets. In each, the web access model defines a structured naming scheme (i.e. URI) to denote computed record sets based on attribute matching patterns. However, the two catalogs do not implement the same naming scheme. In Tagfiler, the naming scheme was tuned for encoding arbitrary graph-query patterns, where one computed set of assets could be derived from another by traversing an arbitrarily chosen linking property.

In ERMrest the relationships between entity types are also captured in the typed schema, corresponding to the underlying RDBMS concept of foreign-key references between tables. ERMrest defines a compact URI naming scheme to traverse such linked entities as a psuedo-hierarchy of related entity sets. A URI denoting one set of typed entities can be extended with the name of another linked entity type to denote a set of related entities of that other type. Either URI may also be extended with filter expressions to denote a subset of entities of the same type.

To see how ERMrest exposes related entities, consider a catalog with entity types *experiment*, *slide*, and *scan* (i.e. image file from a microscope) with simple nesting relationships such that *experiments* may be associated with zero or more *slides* which are associated with zero or more *scans*. The URL:

```
https://bdam.example.org/ermrest/catalog/42/entity/
    experiment/id=123/slide/year=2014/scan
```

is anchored in a particular multi-tenant ERMrest server, selects catalog 42, selects the entity API (for entity access), selects experiments, subsets the experiments by an identifier constraint, selects related slides, subsets the slides by a year constraint, and finally selects related scans.

ERMrest and Tagfiler support complex, ad hoc, declarative query languages in the URL itself by using tokenizers and "look ahead left-to-right" (LALR) parsers normally used to develop new programming languages. We first defined a formal language grammar for the new query languages and then used the Python Lex-Yacc library (PLY; http://www.dabeaz.com/ply/) to generate LALR parsers for the languages. The flexibility of this approach means that the URL scheme (shown in the examples in this section) is not merely a template-based URL pattern but a bona fide declarative query language in its own right. Furthermore, we have avoided the "escape hatch" syndrome in which a native query language (i.e., SPARQL, SQL, etc.) is simply passed as an URL argument or in the message body of a HTTP operation. This results in a true RESTful interface that allows not only HTTP GET but also POST, PUT, and DELETE operations to query, create, update, and delete entries in the catalog, respectively.

With ERMrest, a significant distinction from our earlier Tagfiler approach was that it assists the user with querying across related entities in the system (that is, it simplifies database joins). This is achieved through database introspection. Relational databases such as PostgreSQL, used here, support a standard view called the "information_schema" that allows clients to discover the tables, columns, and foreign key relationships in the database. ERMrest uses this information to automatically detect foreign key relationships that can then be traversed through a pseudo-hierarchical URL, as shown in our above example. For instance, ERMrest can detect that the "scan" table has a foreign key column that references the primary key of the "slide" table. Then, the "syntactic sugar" of the query language is that this relationship can simply be expressed hierarchically in the URL (…slide/<filter>/scan…) without explicitly joining the entities in the filter.

Unlike ERMrest, Tagfiler exposes a triple-like interface for "tagging" assets such as data files and hence was named *Tagfiler*. Tagging represents a compromise between the frequently fluid and evolving nature of human representations and the benefits of strict schema [15] and our initial catalog focused on this highly flexible method of annotation. Use of tags within the catalog were structured by requiring that all tags be defined before use and by providing fine grain access control at the object and attribute level. Tagfiler allows assets to be identified based on patterns constraining arbitrary sets of attributes. Tagfiler is tuned for sparse data by using a Decompositional Storage Model (DSM) [6] to store triples in property-specific tables and to generate complex joining queries when searching. In Tagfiler the type of a metadata record is determined by the properties it has (sometimes referred to as "duck-typed"), with arbitrary combinations of properties allowed on each resource.

To denote the same set of scans in a Tagfiler catalog, consider a catalog where the same three entity types are represented by tagging them with properties to indicate their relationships and local properties. The admittedly cumbersome graph-query URL:

```
https://bdam.example.org/tagfiler/catalog/42/subject/
   slideref=
      @(/year=2014;experimentref=@(/id=123))
      (id;year;fileurl;slideref)
```

is anchored in a multi-tenant Tagfiler server, selects catalog 42, selects the subject API (for graph subject access), and selects subjects tagged with "slideref" referencing other subjects matching a subquery which is wrapped inside "@(...)" and reuses the same search path notation as the subject API. Since Tagfiler subjects are duck-typed, the end of the URL must specify a list of desired scan properties to return (id, year, fileurl, and slideref). The first subquery denotes a set of subjects tagged with "year" 2014 and "experimentref" referencing other subjects matching a second nested subquery. The second subquery denotes a subject with a identifier 123.

The complexity of mapping idiomatic conceptual hierarchies to a Tagfiler graph-query was the motivation for ERMrest's type-aware URL scheme. By being aware of entity types, ERMrest is able to choose the reference and response properties automatically; ERMrest can also follow references in either direction, e.g. given a specific scan it can find the corresponding experiment as:

```
https://bdam.example.org/ermrest/catalog/42/entity/scan/i
d=456/slide/experiment.
```

For complex models with multiple possible reference paths between the same entity types, ERMrest also supports other more verbose URL schemes where a desired reference path is selected explicitly. Thus, the model aware resolution scheme permits idiomatic URLs for typically simple models, while still being able to adapt to complex domain models when necessary.

4.3   Metadata Ingest

There are significant challenges to gaining wide adoption of data repositories [16]. Manual metadata entry is among the most significant barriers to creating data repositories, as it places too much burden on researchers, and is time consuming and error prone. As noted by Plale et al [7], metadata entry into an institutional repository must place a minimal overhead on researchers' time and effort, and must be able to support the wide variety of heterogeneous data, which certainly applies to life sciences.

The two dominant methods for automatically populating metadata catalogs are known as metadata *extraction* and *harvesting* [17]. Metadata harvesting is the approach to generating metadata by inspecting source data for known metadata fields, which may be found in file format headers, such as NIfTI data format headers for Neuroimaging, or interleaved throughout files, such as comment fields in Variable Call Format (VCF) files for genomics. Harvesting methods are assisted by human experts and authors, for instance on the web this is achieved through the usage of META tags in HTML documents, but it applies equally to the well-defined metadata fields of biomedical data formats. The Open Archives Initiative (OAI) has proposed a standard protocol for metadata harvesting (OAI-PMH) [18] in order to support institutional repositories. Metadata extraction, on the other hand, uses algorithmic methods that analyze the contents of files to automatically generate metadata. Research has also shown the efficacy of using automated extraction methods to assist human experts and authors in extracting metadata from data sources [19].

We believe that a blending of these techniques will be most effective for biomedical data, since data sources in this domain are often unstructured or semi-structured. Motivating our approach, we note the following characteristics (see Section 5 for more details on application experiences): the data are not altered once created (i.e. instruments create the primary data which are not edited after creation), the data are stored as flat files and do not support query interfaces (file formats as noted, and occasionally XML repositories), metadata comprise a small subset of the data files (e.g. a 10GB image file may contain only 10KB of metadata), and new files are incrementally added to the system (e.g. when new subjects are scanned or samples are sequenced) throughout the different phases of projects. For these reasons, our metadata ingest framework operates close to the data sources, incrementally harvests and extracts metadata from source files, and uploads only the transformed metadata to the repository along with links back to the source data.

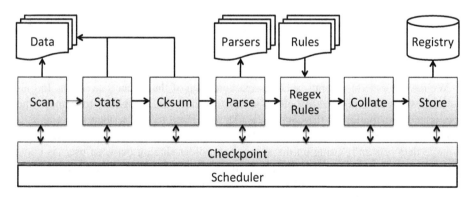

Fig. 2. The ingest pipeline implemented in the IOBox framework. Each processing stage (shown in gray) is checkpointed so that the system can restart efficiently when processing large datasets. Third-party parsers are "plugged into" the framework to support the wide variety of formats for biomedical data. User-defined rules can be specified for transformation during the ingest.

The ingest framework (called IOBox and shown in Fig. 2) includes a series of event-driven stages to integrate data into the catalog and its virtual repository. The IOBox checkpoints the state of the ingest pipeline at each stage in a local, embedded database. The first stage is a file scanning stage that generates a manifest of the source directory. Following the file scan, the IOBox reads basic file statistics, such as the file size, last modified date, etc. New files are then parsed and descriptive metadata extracted.

Biomedical data come in a wide variety of formats with several common formats each for genomics, microscopy, and radiology and many less common formats. The IOBox has a pluggable architecture for integrating third-party parsers, so that the system can be expanded to handle virtually any existing or new file format. Presently, we have developed adapters for HDF5, NetCDF, DICOM, NIfTI, Microsoft Excel, proprietary image formats including Olympus SVI, Aperio SVS, and Hamamatsu NDPI, open microscopy formats OME-XML and OME-TIFF, and text formats such as SAM, VCF, and Comma-Separated Values (CSV) files.

After extracting the raw metadata, the IOBox runs a set of user-defined rules to transform the raw metadata into the user-defined metadata model of the user's BDAM catalog. A rules condition and action are specified using regular expression syntax to allow rules to match a raw metadata field and transform the field into the user model of their catalog. The output of the rules is then collated to associate the metadata fields with the appropriate item in the catalog and then stored in the catalog using the bulk update interface.

4.4   Storage Services

Within BDAM, assets need to be accessed, moved from location to location, and exported for purposes of analysis and publication. Export may involve transformation of the entity, which could range from simple renaming and restructuring of the directory structures, to transcribing the data into a different file format, to combining and transforming the actual data values. Current efforts focus on the simplest of these methods: transfer and renaming.

We have pursued two approaches to manipulation of the actual data assets. Initially, we leveraged a commodity cloud storage service (i.e. Dropbox) to manage the access and distribution of the data assets. The interface to this service is trivial as it transparently replicates locally stored files. However, this service does not scale well to large data sets and setting up the appropriate folder sharing between users is cumbersome. Our current BDAM implementation uses Globus Transfer, a widely used high performance, high-reliability cloud hosted transfer agent [20]. These facilities provide a capability analogous to the consumer experience of using download managers to ensure that data are successfully downloaded from a server to a client machine, retry on transient network failures, and restart at the last transfer checkpoint after an interruption in the download process. Unlike consumer download managers, Globus Transfer has been tuned specifically for moving very large datasets (large volumes of data and/or large numbers of files) over long-haul networks.

4.5   Group Management and Access Control

Throughout the BDAM system, role-based access control policies may be used to grant or restrict access to data, metadata, or to subsets of either. We use Globus Nexus [21] a SaaS identity and group management platform for managing access control in BDAM. These collaboration services (IdP, federation, group management) coupled with fine-grain access control to metadata and data storage services provide the necessary ingredients for creating scientific collaboratories that may span institutional boundaries.

5   Application Experiences

We have applied BDAM configured with both Tagfiler and ERMrest to a number of different use cases. In the following, we provide a high-level overview of some of these with the objective of illustrating how the BDAM concepts have been applied as a means of integrating biomedical digital assets across collaborative projects involving multiple institutions in many cases. These experiences have informed the design and features of the system and allowed us a real-world environment in which to validate our assumptions.

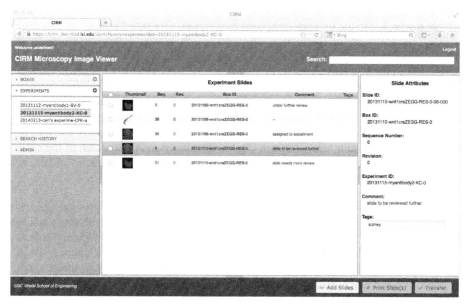

Fig. 3. BDAM solution created for management of digital scans from high-resolution slides scanner at the Center for Regenerative Medicine and Stem Cell Research (CIRM). Left panel provides a browsing interface. The center panel lists the assets that are associated with the selected collection and the right panel displays and enables editing of the attributes of a selected asset.

Center for Regenerative Medicine and Stem Cell Research (CIRM). CIRM operates a microscopy data core with multiple labs sharing slide scanners and networked storage servers. With the acquisition of new high-throughput slide scanners, CIRM was faced with a challenge of creating an integrated view of data from the slides across labs, across different microscopes, and across collaborations that share data beyond the boundaries of the local institute. This environment was typical in that 1) there were no tools available to the researchers, 2) the researchers were being inundated with data and 3) researchers are highly sensitive to any overhead placed on them to document metadata. We have integrated BDAM into their research workflow which includes attaching barcode labels to slides which the slide scanner can read and inserts its contents into metadata within the vendor specific file format as well as encoding it in the scan's file name. Using IOBox the system is able to capture metadata by harvesting data from slide barcodes. A hybrid integration model was developed in which a predefined ERMrest model was used to capture the relationship between a slide, scans of that slide from different microscopes and specific experiments that use those slides while schema editing elements of the BDAM allows the model to be extended with experiment specific attributes. A user interface modeled after familiar photo management solutions (Fig. 3) was developed to minimize the startup overhead. Deployment of the BDAM is in its early phases, however, the response to date from the scientists has been very positive.

USC Physical Sciences Oncology Center (USC PSOC). USC PSOC performs multi-scale research into the biology and physics of cancer. Our data catalog and repository were used to support collection, discovery, and reuse of data products from disparate research teams involving genetics, proteomics, in vitro and in vivo experiments, and computer simulation [22]. The kinds of data products collected include spreadsheets, text and binary files from various instruments, multiple microscopy and gross anatomical image formats, and derived byproducts such as animations, charts, and papers. Several forms of data collection were used including browser-based data submission and automatic replication of content added to shared Dropbox file repositories. A browser-based, faceted search UI was developed to allow search of the catalog by basic metadata properties such as the researcher involved, the kind of file, or the cancer cell-line or drugs being tested in the experiment.

Doheny Eye Institute's Image Reading Center (DIRC). DIRC provides expert ophthalmic image evaluation in support of clinical trials. Our RESTful data catalog and repository was augmented with a browser-based GUI agent to securely collect imaging studies from internationally distributed ophthalmology clinics, annotate them with trial study metadata, and track studies through a workflow involving image quality assurance and diagnostic grading. Two integration modes were explored: a browser-based GUI to securely download data sets from the repository to an imaging workstation, and a local trial management system configured to automatically retrieve study metadata and images using the RESTful API. Role-based access control was used to protect image and metadata confidentiality and integrity, providing write-once capability to submitting clinics and limited read-only access to studies for only the original submitting clinic and the appropriate DIRC staff.

Leonard D. Schaeffer Center for Health Policy and Economics. The Schaeffer Center conducts econometric analyses on a variety of data sets representing health events over large populations of patients. Due to the scope and complexity of the data sets, the analyses often involve a large number of files and non-trivial data storage resources. Tagfiler was used to store an index of a data and program library containing hundreds of thousands of files. This index was populated by IOBox using a set of heuristic annotation rules to extract metadata from deeply structured file path names. A browser-based, faceted search UI was used to allow search of the index by basic metadata properties such as the researcher involved, the kind of file content, the project or source dataset involved, and file metadata such as ownership, size, and timestamp information. After ingest, bulk update operations were used to further organize data by domain specific concepts such as source of the data, disease type, etc.

6 Discussion

The schema-neutral nature of our system made it easier to adjust the metadata scope on the fly, allowing incremental refinement of metadata within a catalog. Very heterogeneous data assets can be tracked, reducing the metadata on those assets to a core set of opaque file-container attributes. However, user investment is necessary to augment this with enough descriptive metadata to support data discovery. In projects where data-producing users did not see the value in this investment, the minimalist metadata was not sufficient to support discovery. Instead, potential collaborators had to be identified by other human processes and directed to coordinate with one another; in those cases, the BDAM approach was still useful to archive content or facilitate transfer of large files.

We often encounter user communities who specify semantic web standards such as RDF as one of their feature requirements. However, in our data sharing pilot studies, we found that most users actually did not find triple-based metadata to be intuitive nor practical. The most common reasons they identified for requesting RDF were that: 1) they had heard of an ontology specific to their domain that might be useful, 2) they had heard the idea of a shared ontology and liked the idea of shared vocabulary in general, 3) they had been told that RDF was the way to make data interoperable, D) they believed RDF was more flexible than SQL in allowing schema change.

In our experience, most non-computer scientist data users seem to find it easier to think about entity-relational models; most importantly, they can start with naive understanding of flat tables, and only learn more sophisticated concepts such as typing, keys, and references later as their understanding of the problem develops. As Tagfiler evolved, we found the table-like access APIs to be the most embraced capability, and indeed we found it easiest to explain it to users as a catalog containing "one large, wide table" where the user did not have to be worried about lots of missing values in a particular row. We also had users asking for more SQL-like constraints so that they could enforce certain data structuring conventions in a community catalog. Our shift to explicit entity-relational models in ERMrest is largely motivated by these observations.

7   Future Work

There are a number of directions we hope to take BDAM in the future. These include:

Optimized Storage. Our web services catalog interfaces place a clean separation between the service model and the underlying storage model used to store the descriptive metadata. We plan to provide mechanisms that will support a hybrid storage model that supports both the decomposed storage optimized for sparse representations with the dense table oriented model that is better suited for more dense descriptive element

Improved User Interfaces. To date, we have explored two classes of generic interface: a facet based search and the three-pane interface used by CIRM. Both of which require some significant configuration prior to use in a specific application. However, the web services based introspection interface in the BDAM catalog makes it possible to perform a significant amount of auto configuration

Data Extraction and Analytics Integration. Current BDAM file management can only perform simple renaming operations. In general, we will require more extensive file consolidation, extraction and transformation operations. Of specific interest is providing the extraction methods and interfaces necessary to hand data assets off to external tools and used for biomedical data analysis and general purpose analytic frameworks.

8   Conclusions

The lack of tools to help researchers in the life sciences integrate, organize and manage their data is a significant gap that has significant impact on productivity and reliability. Taking a cue from widely used systems in the consumer space, a biomedical digital asset management system can close this gap, providing a platform for integrating data from multiple sources and integrating that data into the daily workflow associated with discovery in the life sciences. By focusing on ease of use and low barrier to entry via automated methods delivery via software as a service mechanisms, end users will both use and benefit from a BDAM approach to integration.

Acknowledgments. The authors would like to acknowledge the contributions of Serban Voinea in implementing the Tagfiler catalog and several of the use cases and Ian Foster, Kyle Chard for their fruitful discussions on many of the topics presented in this paper.

References

1. Howe, B., Cole, G., Souroush, E., Koutris, P., Key, A., Khoussainova, N., Battle, L.: Database-as-a-Service for Long-Tail Science. In: Bayard Cushing, J., French, J., Bowers, S. (eds.) SSDBM 2011. LNCS, vol. 6809, pp. 480–489. Springer, Heidelberg (2011)

2. Halevy, A., Franklin, M., Maier, D.: Principles of Dataspace Systems. In: PODS 2006. ACM, Chicago (2006)
3. Digital Asset Management. Wikipedia (2014)
4. Tunkelang, D.: Faceted Search. Synthesis Lectures on Information Concepts, Retrieval, and Services, vol. 1, pp. 1–80 (2009)
5. Halevy, A., Rajaraman, A., Ordille, J.: Data integration: the teenage years. In: VLDB 2006, pp. 9–16. VLDB Endowment, Seoul (2006)
6. Corwin, J., et al.: Dynamic tables: An architecture for managing evolving, heterogeneous biomedical data in relational database management systems. Journal of the American 14, 86–93 (2007)
7. Plale, B., et al.: SEAD Virtual Archive: Building a Federation of Institutional Repositories for Long-Term Data Preservation in Sustainability Science. International Journal of Digital Curation 8, 172–180 (2013)
8. Hellerstein, J.M., et al.: The MADlib analytics library: or MAD skills, the SQL. In: Proceedings of the VLDB Endowment, pp. 1700–1711 (2012)
9. Smith, M., et al.: DSpace: An Open Source Dynamic Digital Repository. D-Lib Magazine 9 (2003)
10. Singh, G., et al.: A Metadata Catalog Service for Data Intensive Applications. In: Super-Computing (SC 2003). ACM, Phoenix (2003)
11. Marcus, D.S., et al.: The Extensible Neuroimaging Archive Toolkit: an informatics platform for managing, exploring, and sharing neuroimaging data. Neuroinformatics 5, 11–34 (2007)
12. Shoshani, A., Sim, A., Gu, J.: Storage resource managers: Middleware components for grid storage. In: NASA Conference Publication, pp. 209–224 (2002)
13. Rajasekar, A., et al.: iRODS Primer: Integrated Rule-Oriented Data System. Synthesis Lectures on Information Concepts, Retrieval, and Services, vol. 2, pp. 1–143 (2010)
14. Bittman, T.: Mind the Gap: Here Comes the Hybrid Cloud. In: Gartner Blog Network (2012)
15. Cattuto, C., Loreto, V., Pietronero, L.: Semiotic dynamics and collaborative tagging. Proceedings of the National Academy of Sciences 104(5), 1461–1464 (2007)
16. Davis, P.M., Connolly, M.J.L.: Institutional Repositories: Evaluating the Reasons for Non-use of Cornell University's Installation of DSpace. D-Lib Magazine 13 (2007)
17. Greenberg, J.: Metadata Extraction and Harvesting: A Comparison of Two Automatic Metadata Generation Applications. Journal of Internet Cataloging 6, 59–82 (2004)
18. Lagoze, C., de Sompel, H.: The making of the open archives initiative protocol for metadata harvesting. Library hi tech 21, 118–128 (2003)
19. Tuchinda, R., Szekely, P., Knoblock, C.A.: Building data integration queries by demonstration. In: Proceedings of the 12th International Conference on Intelligent User Interfaces - IUI 2007, p. 170. ACM Press, New York (2007)
20. Allen, B., et al.: Software as a service for data scientists. Communications of the ACM 55, 81 (2012)
21. Ananthakrishnan, R., et al.: Globus Nexus: An identity, profile, and group management platform for science gateways and other collaborative science applications. In: 2013 IEEE International Conference on Cluster Computing (CLUSTER), pp. 1–3 (2013)
22. Agus, D.B., et al.: A physical sciences network characterization of non-tumorigenic and metastatic cells. Scientific Reports 3, 1449 (2013)

Mining Linked Open Data:
A Case Study with Genes Responsible
for Intellectual Disability

Gabin Personeni[1], Simon Daget[1], Céline Bonnet[2,3], Philippe Jonveaux[2,3],
Marie-Dominique Devignes[1], Malika Smaïl-Tabbone[1], and Adrien Coulet[1]

[1] LORIA (CNRS, Inria NGE, Université de Lorraine),
Campus Scientifique, Vandoeuvre-lès-Nancy, F-54506, France
[2] Laboratoire de Génétique Médicale, Centre Hospitalier Universitaire de Nancy,
Vandoeuvre-lès-Nancy, France
[3] INSERM U-954, Université de Lorraine, Rue du Morvan,
Vandoeuvre-lès-Nancy, France

Abstract. Linked Open Data (LOD) constitute a unique dataset that
is in a standard format, partially integrated, and facilitates connections
with domain knowledge represented within semantic web ontologies. Increasing amounts of biomedical data provided as LOD consequently offer
novel opportunities for knowledge discovery in biomedicine. However,
most data mining methods are neither adapted to LOD format, nor
adapted to consider domain knowledge. We propose in this paper an
approach for selecting, integrating, and mining LOD with the goal of
discovering genes responsible for a disease. The selection step relies on a
set of choices made by a domain expert to isolate relevant pieces of LOD.
Because these pieces are potentially not linked, an integration step is required to connect unlinked pieces. The resulting graph is subsequently
mined using Inductive Logic Programming (ILP) that presents two main
advantages. First, the input format compliant with ILP is close to the
format of LOD. Second, domain knowledge can be added to this input
and considered by ILP. We have implemented and applied this approach
to the characterization of genes responsible for intellectual disability. On
the basis of this real-world use case, we present an evaluation of our mining approach and discuss its advantages and drawbacks for the mining
of biomedical LOD.

1 Introduction

Linked Open Data (LOD) are part of a community effort to build a semantic
web, where web resources can be interpreted both by humans and machines.
LOD are available as a large and growing collection of datasets represented in a
standard format (that includes the use of RDF and URIs), partially connected to
each other and to domain knowledge represented within semantic web ontologies
[1]. For these reasons, LOD offer novel opportunities for the development of
successful data integration and knowledge discovery approaches.

H. Galhardas and E. Rahm (Eds.): DILS 2014, LNBI 8574, pp. 16–31, 2014.
© Springer International Publishing Switzerland 2014

This recent availability of LOD can be particularly beneficial to the life sciences, where relevant data are spread over various data resources with no agreement on a unique representation of biological entities [2]. Consequently, data integration is an initial challenge one faces if one wants to mine life science data considering several data sources. Various initiatives such as Bio2RDF, LOD drug data, PDBj or the EBI platform aim at pushing life sciences data into the LOD cloud with the idea of facilitating their integration [3, 4, 5, 6]. It results from these initiatives a large collection of life-science data unequally connected but in a standard format and available for mining.

In addition to their integrated dimension, LOD may be connected to domain knowledge represented within ontologies such as the Gene Ontology [7]. Ontologies provide a formal representation of a particular domain that can be used to support automatic reasoning. We have investigated that ontologies and their associated reasoning mechanisms can be coupled with data mining to facilitate the process of knowledge discovery [8, 9]. We would like to extend this investigation to the context of LOD. Despite good will and emerging standard practices for publishing data as LOD, several drawbacks make their use still challenging [10, 11]. Among existing difficulties we can list the limited amount of links between datasets, the lack of update on published datasets, the variety of SPARQL versions supported by systems that enable querying LOD.

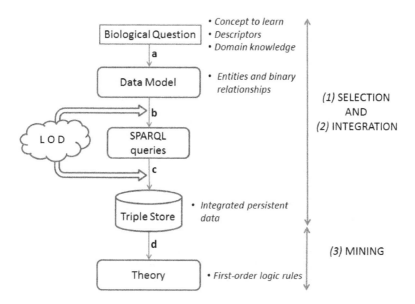

Fig. 1. Outline of the methodology used for preparing and mining Linked Open Data (LOD). *a*: Conceptualization in term of entities and binary relationships; *b*: Mapping onto various LOD datasets; *c*: Retrieval of triples using SPARQL queries; *d*: Relational learning with Inductive Logic Programming (ILP).

We propose here an approach that is schematized in Figure 1 and that enables to *(1)* select, *(2)* integrate and then *(3)* mine LOD with Inductive Logic Programming (ILP). *(1)* The selection of LOD is achieved with respect to a conceptualization of data related to a biomedical question. This conceptualization is driven by a biomedical expert and, in this paper, is motivated by our will to characterize genes responsible for intellectual disability. *(2)* The integration of LOD is made possible both by the use of links present in LOD and by the manual definition of mappings between our conceptualization and LOD. Links and mappings enable to automatically build SPARQL queries and subsequently retrieve LOD triples to mine. In addition, our mappings enable the generation of unpublished links between LOD entities, consequently contributing to the community effort. *(3)* Finally, triples are mined using ILP that is particularly adapted to the format of LOD and capable of taking into account domain knowledge defined in ontologies.

The next section presents a state of the art of data mining applied to LOD and introduces ILP. The third section presents the LOD selection and integration made in preparation for the mining. The fourth section reports about mining experiments with ILP on selected triples. The last section concludes on experiments and presents perspectives of this initial work.

2   State of the Art

2.1   Preparing LOD for Mining

The complexity of LOD has motivated several studies about the preparation (*i.e.*, selection, integration, formatting) of data before mining. For instance, we proposed a system that guides the selection of LOD by structuring data within a lattice that provides insight about which type of entities are related and how [12]. Callahan *et al.* proposed to map LOD from various datasets to an upper-level ontology named SIO. This ontology serves consequently as a global schema and its terms are used to write federated queries over LOD datasets [13]. SADI is a general framework to facilitate the discovery and use of web services [14]. Because it has been developed with semantic web technologies, SADI is well adapted to define pipelines that can query SPARQL endpoints and integrate their results. The COEUS platform follows a similar rationale but includes a federation layer that facilitates data integration [15].

Any of these solutions is well adapted when either entities have a unique URI over distinct datasets, or when links have been defined between datasets. Unfortunately, these two prerequisites are not guaranteed in LOD. In this work, we want to be able to use any LOD dataset, even if this requires to define novel mappings between datasets, using various types of relationships. For this reason we propose a simple but generic way for selecting and integrating LOD to be mined.

2.2 Mining LOD

The emergence of several workshops about the mining of LOD illustrates the rise of interest for this topic, both in the semantic web and data mining communities. A first type of contribution in this domain aims at completing or correcting the LOD. In that vein, Gangemi *et al.* proposed an approach to type systematically DBpedia entities using graph patterns and disambiguation techniques [16]. Other authors studied how to propose systematically missing links, particularly between unrelated datasets [17, 18]. For example, Brenninkmeijer *et al.* developed a tool for proposing `owl:sameAs` links between unrelated drugs of LOD datasets [19].

A second group of works explores how some peculiarities of LOD can help data mining. For example, Percha *et al.* used paths between distinct drugs in linked data to predict novel drug-drug interactions [20]. Here, the fact that relationships and entities are typed in LOD enable to define features that characterise possible paths between drugs and consequently to train a random forest classifier. Pathak *et al.* proposed a study on how federated queries over Electronic Health Records and drug related LOD could enable the discovery of novel drug-drug interactions [21].

To our knowledge, only few seminal works have explored how LOD mining can take advantages of knowledge representation [22, 23]. In this work we propose to explore this direction using ILP.

2.3 Inductive Logic Programming

ILP Principles. Inductive Logic Programming (ILP) allows us to learn a concept definition from observations, *i.e.*, a set of positive examples $(E+)$ and a set of negative examples $(E-)$, and background knowledge (B) [24]. Given $E+$, $E-$, and B the goal is to induce a set of rules or a theory T that is consistent ($T \cup B$ covers or explains each positive example), and complete ($T \cup B$ does not cover any negative example). In most ILP systems both B and T are represented as definite clauses (or prolog programs) in first-order logic, *i.e.*, a disjunction of literals with one positive literal. A rule has the form "head :- body" and is interpreted as: if the conditions in the body are true then the head is true as a logical consequence. The background knowledge B includes the relational description of the examples using a set of relevant n-ary predicates such as

protein_mf('gpaC', 'receptor binding').

which expresses the fact that the GO (Gene Ontology) term 'receptor binding' is one of the molecular functions of the protein 'gpaC' (with respect to the annotation database GOA). B also includes a priori domain knowledge, *i.e.*, a set of facts and rules which do not refer to any example but express what is known about the elements which describe the examples. For instance, the fact

subClass('insulin receptor binding', 'receptor binding').

expresses a *is-a* semantic relationship between two GO terms. Moreover, the following inference rule[1] expresses the transitivity of the subClass binary predicate:

$$\texttt{subClass}(X, Z) \; :- \; \texttt{subClass}(X, Y), \; \texttt{subClass}(Y, Z).$$

The theory T is a set of rules which cover as many positive examples as possible and the fewest negative examples. The head of each rule is the concept to learn whereas the body contains the induced description of the concept (based on a generalization of examples). An example of a rule when studying genes responsible for a disease has the form

$$\texttt{is\_responsible}(X) \; :- \; \texttt{gene\_protein}(X, Y), \; \texttt{protein\_mf}(Y, \text{'receptor binding'}).$$

which expresses that if the gene X produces a protein Y and Y has 'receptor binding' as a molecular function then X is responsible for the studied disease.

The rule search is performed in a clause space where the clause subsumption allows building generalizations or specializations of the clauses [25]. As the clause space is too large to be exhaustively explored, heuristic mechanisms exist to reduce its size. These mechanisms (called learning biases) allow the user to define which kind of rules (s)he wants to get by setting some parameters that influence the rule search strategy.

The Aleph Program. The experiments reported in this paper were conducted with the Aleph program whose basic algorithm is described in four steps [26]:

- Select a seed example to be generalized. If none exists, stop.
- Construct the most specific clause that entails the example selected, and is compliant with the language restrictions provided. This clause is called the "bottom clause".
- Find a clause more general than the bottom clause. This is done by searching for some subset of the literals in the bottom clause that has the "best" evaluation score.
- The clause with the best score is added as a rule to the current theory, and all examples made redundant are removed. Return to Step 1.

Several parameters can be set for tuning the theory construction. For instance, the rule evaluation function can be chosen and the default one is based on the difference between the number of covered positive examples and the number of covered negative examples. The noise parameter is the maximum number of negative examples that an acceptable rule may cover (default value is 0). This parameter can be set to higher values in case of noisy data. The min-pos parameter is the minimal number of positive examples that a rule must cover.

---

[1] In the Prolog syntax, terms starting with an uppercase letter are variables.

3 LOD Selection and Integration

3.1 Conceptualization

In our approach, the first step is to build an entity-relationship (ER) model decribing the entities to consider for a given study. The goal of the ER model is to provide an abstract model of data that are relevant to mine. This step is realized with an expert of the domain, and does not require any knowledge of what data is available in LOD and how it is structured. An ER model consists of a conceptualization usually made of entities, relationships and attributes. We use only a subset of those: entities and binary relationships without attributes (similarly to RDF properties). In our case, n-ary relationships and relationships with attributes are represented with a composition of binary relationships using the reification mechanism. Figure 2 presents the ER model defined for our study of genes responsible for Intellectual Disability (ID).

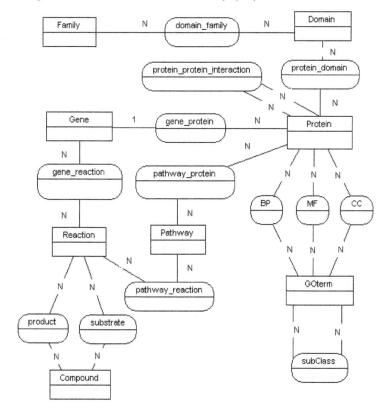

Fig. 2. Entity-relationship (ER) model of data on genes responsible for Intellectual Disability (ID). For the sake of clarity, we have not represented gene location, which is composed of chromosome, arm, region, band, sub-band and sub-sub-band. BP, MF and CC represent GO-term annotations of proteins (Biological Process, Molecular Function and Cellular Component annotations respectively).

Table 1. Sources and count of distinct collected individuals that instantiate each entity of our ER model

Entity	SPARQL endpoint	#Individuals
Gene	`cu.gene.bio2rdf.org/sparql` `cu.kegg.bio2rdf.org/sparql`	549
Protein	`beta.sparql.uniprot.org/sparql`	1257
Pathway	`cu.kegg.bio2rdf.org/sparql` `www.ebi.ac.uk/rdf/services/reactome/sparql`	580
Reaction	`cu.kegg.bio2rdf.org/sparql`	433
Compound	`cu.kegg.bio2rdf.org/sparql`	628
GOterm	`cu.goa.bio2rdf.org/sparql` `sparql.bioontology.org/sparql`	7770
Domain	`cu.interpro.bio2rdf.org/sparql`	262
Family	`cu.interpro.bio2rdf.org/sparql`	781
	Total	12260

3.2   Mapping the ER Model onto LOD and Individual Identification

Mapping Definition. LOD integration consists primarily in mapping our expert-defined ER model onto LOD types of entities and of relationships. This mapping is materialized by defining correspondances between each entity of the model and one or many RDF entity types of LOD; and between each relationship of the model and RDF properties present in LOD. Indeed, distinct LOD datasets may use distinct entity types to refer to a single entity of our model. For instance, the entity `Gene` of the model is mapped to two entity types: `<http://bio2rdf.org/geneid:vocabulary:Gene>` and `http://bio2rdf.org/kegg_vocabulary:Gene` respectively used in two datasets of Bio2RDF: NCBI Gene and KEGG. Each entity is further defined by a *concept definition* that can be either an RDF entity type, its negation, the domain/range of a property, or the union/intersection of two entity types. Similarly, the relationships of the ER model can be mapped to one property or a composition of properties (or inverse properties), or to an artificial property subsuming them. For instance, the relationship `gene_reaction` between a gene and a reaction (which represents the fact that the gene produces an enzyme that catalyzes the reaction) can be mapped to `kegg:xGene⁻ ∘ kegg:xEnzyme⁻`.[2] Table 1 and Table 2 list entities and relationships of our ER model and the datasets they are mapped to.

Individual Identification. Because the mapping can associate one entity with several datasets, it can cause redundancy. To guarantee the consistency of data related by our mapping, we need additional information on individual identity.

---

[2] The property `kegg:xGene` relates genes to enzymes and `kegg:xEnzyme` relates enzymes to reactions, whereas `gene_reaction` relates directly reactions to genes. The latter is a composition (denoted by ∘) of the inverses (denoted by ⁻) of `kegg:xEnzyme` and `kegg:xGene`.

Table 2. Sources and count of distinct collected instances for each relationship of our ER model

Relationship	SPARQL endpoint	#Individuals
gene_protein	beta.sparql.uniprot.org/sparql	819
gene_reaction	cu.kegg.bio2rdf.org/sparql	500
pp_interaction	cu.irefindex.bio2rdf.org/sparql	742
pathway_protein	www.ebi.ac.uk/rdf/services/reactome/sparql	767
protein_domain	cu.interpro.bio2rdf.org/sparql	262
pathway_reaction	cu.interpro.bio2rdf.org/sparql	706
substrate	cu.kegg.bio2rdf.org/sparql	938
product	cu.kegg.bio2rdf.org/sparql	960
protein_bp	cu.goa.bio2rdf.org/sparql	10242
protein_cc	cu.goa.bio2rdf.org/sparql	4358
protein_mf	cu.goa.bio2rdf.org/sparql	4063
subClass	sparql.bioontology.org/sparql	12779
domain_family	cu.interpro.bio2rdf.org/sparql	1238
gene_chromosome	cu.gene.bio2rdf.org/sparql	538
gene_chromosome_arm	cu.gene.bio2rdf.org/sparql	538
gene_chromosome_region	cu.gene.bio2rdf.org/sparql	538
gene_chromosome_band	cu.gene.bio2rdf.org/sparql	538
gene_chromosome_subband	cu.gene.bio2rdf.org/sparql	311
gene_chromosome_subsubband	cu.gene.bio2rdf.org/sparql	63
	Total	40900

Individuals are identified in LOD by their URIs. The main issue in mining LOD from several datasets is that two distinct URIs from different LOD datasets may refer to the same real world object. Individuals' URIs links from one LOD dataset to another may be available, ideally using the property owl:sameAs, although sometimes a less precise link, such as rdfs:seeAlso or a dataset dependent predicate is used. For entity types that mapped onto several LOD datasets, an automatic way of resolving identity of individuals needs to be established. In our case study, this is achieved through several means:

- Using when available in LOD, links that express equivalence between alternative URIs of an individual, such as rdfs:seeAlso.
- Using LOD features associated with individuals to assess the identity:
  - URIs themselves sometimes embed enough data to assess that two individuals are identical. For example, in some datasets, gene URIs contain the NCBI Gene ID: the human gene with Gene ID 5091 is represented by the URI <http://bio2rdf.org/geneid:5091> in Bio2RDF NCBI Gene, and <http://bio2rdf.org/kegg_vocabulary:hsa:5091> in Bio2RDF KEGG. An obvious link between the two URIs can be made on the basis of the Gene ID.
  - Individuals can be associated with literals that identify them across datasets, such as the HGNC gene symbol for genes, that is used to identify genes in Bio2RDF NCBI Gene and Bio2RDF OMIM datasets.

Using these methods, given a URI in a given dataset, we can find the corresponding URI in another dataset. Links we generated this way are available at `http://www.loria.fr/~coulet/dils14/individual_identities.html`. More sophisticated methods based on URIs or literals can be designed to compute identity.

3.3   Triple Retrieval and Storage

For the purpose of ILP mining, a set of positive examples and a set of negative examples must be provided. In our study, positives examples are genes responsible for Intellectual Disability (ID), while negative examples are genes that are not responsible for this type of disease. Positive examples were selected from a state-of-the-art study about genes responsible for ID by Inlow and Restifo [27]. We selected negative examples among genes responsible for diseases other than ID. To this aim, we first selected phenotypes in OMIM which do not contain ID as a symptom. From this large set of phenotypes, biomedical experts advised the selection of a subset of phenotypes clearly distinct from ID. Genes responsible for these phenotypes were then retrieved from OMIM. The final set of negative examples is selected from stratified sampling with respect to the overall number of genes associated with each phenotype.[3]

Given the ER model and its mapping to LOD entity types and roles, SPARQL queries can be built in a systematic way to retrieve the data from LOD. As an illustration, for building a SPARQL query to retrieve the families of protein domains (`domain_family` relationship in Table 2) the following mapping was used: the `Domain` entity is mapped to the entity type `http://bio2rdf.org/interpro_vocabulary:Domain`; `Family` is mapped to `http://bio2rdf.org/interpro_vocabulary:Family`; and the `domain_family` relationship is mapped to the `<http://bio2rdf.org/interpro_vocabulary:contains>`⁻ property. On this basis, the following query is built:

```
SELECT ?x ?y
WHERE {
   ?x a <http://bio2rdf.org/interpro_vocabulary:Domain>.
   ?y a <http://bio2rdf.org/interpro_vocabulary:Family>.
   ?y <http://bio2rdf.org/interpro_vocabulary:contains> ?x.
   FILTER(?x = ...)
}
```

The `FILTER` statement of the query is used to retrieve only triples associated with genes reponsible/not responsible for ID.

Once the SPARQL queries are generated and executed, then retrieved data is automatically stored in a triple store. Our triple store relies on a simple relational database built upon the ER model. To each entity corresponds a table whose columns are a local identifier and URIs from each dataset mapped to that

---

[3] The two sets of genes are available at `http://www.loria.fr/čoulet/dils14/positives` and `http://www.loria.fr/~coulet/dils14/negatives`.

entity. To each relationship corresponds a table whose columns are the local identifiers of its subject and its object. The number of individuals collected with this method starting from a list of 549 genes (282 positive and 267 negative examples) are indicated in Table 1 and Table 2 (last column). Our method allows to add new entity types and relationships to our model without discarding previously collected data. However, updating collected data is not possible without recollection of all data on a given entity type or relationship.

4 ILP Mining of LOD

4.1 ILP Experiments and Results

The aim of the mining step is to learn by ILP the concept of genes responsible for Intellectual Disability (ID) from the set of integrated triples relative to positive and negative examples of genes. The experiments were conducted with the Aleph program by setting the parameters *rule size, minpos, noise, minacc*[4] respectively to 6, 5, 3 and 85%. The *noise* parameter allows rules to tolerate a few exceptions (negative examples). This constitutes an advantage when dealing with noisy data such as LOD.

The outcome of the mining experiment is used both for predictive and descriptive purposes. The predictive power of the first-order logic (FOL) rules is evaluated by cross-validation whereas their descriptive power is analyzed qualitatively.

Our first experiment ($G1$) applies to the genes and their background knowledge (*i.e.*, proteins, pathways, etc.) including their GO annotations plus their direct parents using the *is-a* relationship (denoted by $\mathtt{subClass_1}$) between GO-terms. Then we wanted to assess the contribution of domain knowledge by allowing 2 to 4 generalization inferences on the *is-a* GO structure, which is a rooted directed acyclic graph. For n generalization steps, we add $2 \times n$ inference rules in the .b file (one of the three inputs of the Aleph program) as follows:

> One inference rule for each i in $2 \ldots n$:
>
> $\quad \mathtt{subClass}_i(\mathtt{X}, \mathtt{Z}) \ \mathtt{:-} \ \mathtt{subClass}_{i-1}(\mathtt{X}, \mathtt{Y}), \ \mathtt{subClass}_1(\mathtt{Y}, \mathtt{Z}).$
>
> One inference rule for each i in $1 \ldots n$:
>
> $\quad \mathtt{subClass}(\mathtt{X}, \mathtt{Y}) \ \mathtt{:-} \ \mathtt{subClass}_i(\mathtt{X}, \mathtt{Y}).$
>
> One rule expressing the reflexivity of the $\mathtt{subClass}$ relationship :
>
> $\quad \mathtt{subClass}(\mathtt{X}, \mathtt{X}) \ \mathtt{:-} \ \mathtt{goterm}(\mathtt{X}).$

In this study the mining experiment was executed with n varying from 1 to 4, leading to a maximum of 1 ($G1$ experiment), 2 ($G2$ experiment), 3 ($G3$ experiment), and 4 ($G4$ experiment) generalization steps respectively. Examination of the resulting 4 theories revealed that the produced rules mostly contain

---

[4] The *minacc* parameter is the minimum ratio of positives examples among the covered examples.

predicates related to GO-terms. Other predicates representing pathways or interactions between proteins occur very rarely. This can be explained by the fact that GO annotations are plethoric compared to data on pathways, protein domains or protein-protein interactions. This motivated us to run a fifth experiment (named $no - GO$) for analyzing all predicates excepting the GO-term facts. Complete theories produced in the five experiments are accessible online at `http://www.loria.fr/~coulet/dils14/theories.pdf`. Table 3 shows several metrics calculated for monitoring the effect of adding GO-term facts and increasing the number of generalization steps. The number of rules in the theory

Table 3. Statistics on the theories produced by our five experiments. avg/max/min pos covered: Average/maximum/minimum number of positive examples covered by the rules of each theory.

Experiment	#rules	avg pos covered	max pos covered	min pos covered
$no - GO$	11	8.4	15	5
$G1$	22	14	35	6
$G2$	19	15.5	38	6
$G3$	18	15.1	39	6
$G4$	16	16.2	42	5

doubles when adding GO-term facts (from $no-GO$ to $G1$) and the average number of covered examples increases from 8.4 to 14, with its maximum increasing from 15 to 35. This indicates that GO-term facts play a very positive role in the ILP process during learning. As the number of generalization steps increases from 1 to 4 the number of rules decreases (from 22 to 16) whereas the average number of covered examples slightly increases from 14 to 16.2, with a increase of the maximum (from 35 to 42). These results confirm the intuition that with more generalization steps, theories tend to become more compact with fewer rules, each of them covering more examples. However it is important at that stage to assess the predictive power of each theory.

4.2   Evaluation of the Results

We evaluate the outcome of the mining step from a predictive point of view using cross-validation. Dedicated Knime workflows were used for that purpose [28, 29]. During cross-validation, a gene is predicted as responsible for ID if it is covered by at least one rule of the theory. Otherwise, it is predicted as not responsible for ID.

Table 4 reports the results of the leave-one-out cross-validation of ILP learning for the experiments $no - GO$ and $G1$ to $G4$. The results show that without GO-term facts ($no - GO$), the prediction accuracy is rather low (59.6%) with a high specificity but a very low sensitivity. When using GO-terms the prediction indicators are better. They improve up to an accuracy of 69.8% as we allow Aleph to use more domain knowledge (by performing more generalizations). As it is difficult to provide comparative results, we continue with a qualitative analysis of our results.

Table 4. Results of the leave-one-out cross-validation the theories produced by the 5 experiments. TP/FP: True/False Positives, TN/FN: True/False Negatives, Sens.: Sensitivity, Spec.: Specificity, Acc: Accuracy.

Experiment	TP	FP	TN	FN	Sens.(%)	Spec.(%)	Acc.(%)
$no - GO$	75	15	**252**	207	26.6	**94.4**	59.6
$G1$	135	50	217	147	47.9	81.3	64.1
$G2$	157	52	215	125	55.7	80.5	67.8
$G3$	157	49	218	125	55.7	81.7	68.3
$G4$	**161**	45	222	**121**	**57.1**	83.1	**69.8**

Table 5. Right parts of the rules of the $no - GO$ theory, followed by, respectively, the number of positive and negative examples covered by that rule

#	Right part of rule		
1	gene_in_reaction(A, 'Ubiquinol+Acceptor⇔Ubiquinone+Reduced Acceptor').	7	0
2	gene_in_reaction(A, B), gene_protein(A, C), pp_interaction(C,D), pp_interaction(D, C).	6	0
3	gene_in_reaction(A, B), gene_protein(A, C), pp_interaction(C, P30480).	7	0
4	gene_in_reaction(A, B), gene_ch(A, '1')	14	0
5	gene_in_reaction(A, B), gene_ch(A, x)	15	2
6	gene_in_pathway(A, 'Alanine and aspartate metabolism').	6	1
7	gene_in_pathway(A, 'Valine, leucine and isoleucine degradation').	11	1
8	gene_chromosome_band(A, '22q13').	6	0
9	gene_in_pathway(A, 'N-Glycan biosynthesis').	8	0
10	gene_in_pathway(A, 'Formation of TC-NER repair complex').	5	0
11	gene_in_pathway(A, 'Glycosaminoglycan degradation').	8	0

4.3   Qualitative Analysis and Discussion

We analyze here the obtained theories from the descriptive point of view, *i.e.*, how well do the rules characterize genes responsible for ID? Table 5 shows the rules obtained from the $no - GO$ experiment: in the absence of GO-term facts ($no - GO$ experiment), we observe several rules containing predicates related to chromosomal localization such as rule 4 and 5 pointing to chromosomes 1 and X as possible reservoirs of genes for ID. In addition, rule 8 points to a more constrained location on chromosome 22. Other rules contain the gene_in_pathway predicate (rules 6, 7, 9, 10, 11) in which one can mostly recognize pathways involved in the metabolism of the cell. Indeed inherited metabolic disorders are considered as an important etiology for ID [30].

In the presence of GO-term facts (experiments $G1$ to $G4$), the repertoire of GO-terms appearing in the rules either as direct protein annotation or as common ancestor after generalization varies with the experiment and the generalization degree. In total we counted 47, 7 and 14 distinct GO-terms pertainining from the Biological Process (BP), Molecular Function (MF) and Cellular Component (CC) aspects of the GO ontology respectively. Among the BP-terms of GO we could again recognize terms describing metabolic processes of the cell, but also terms related to gene expression mechanisms and to nervous system development which make sense when dealing with ID. Interesting rules are combining `protein_bp` and `protein_mf` predicates such as rule 16 in the $G4$ theory:

is_responsible(A) :- gene_protein(A, B), protein_mf(B, C),

                    subClass(C, 'ion binding'),

                    protein_bp(B, 'carbohydrate metabolic process').

Such rules suggest that the descriptive power of the theories increases when domain knowledge is taken into account. The value of adding generalization can be illustrated on rules having `subClass` terms concerning 'organonitrogen compound metabolism'. Rules 3 from $G1$ and 7 from $G2$ theories both contain the subClass(C, 'organonitrogen compound **metabolic** process') term and each of them covers 23 positive examples. Rules 4 from $G3$ and 4 from $G4$ theories both contain the subClass(C, 'organonitrogen compound **catabolic** process') term which refers to a more specific GO-term than in $G1$ and $G2$ ('catabolism' is one aspect of 'metabolism') but these rules cover 39 positive examples in the $G3$ and 42 positive examples in the $G4$ theories. Thus allowing for more generalization steps has helped to increase the coverage of the rule but also to better specify the feature shared by the positive examples. Several other examples similar to this one are found across the $G1$ to $G4$ theories.

5   Conclusion and Perspectives

This paper proposes an original approach for selecting, integrating and mining LOD, successfully applied to a real-world use case in the life sciences. The results confirm that ILP is adapted to the LOD context and actually allows to exploit biological ontologies available in LOD. Both quantitative and qualitative analyses show promising results. Obtained theories display high specificity, thus limiting the amount of false positives. Each rule characterizes a significant subset of positive genes (16 on average for the best theory). This illustrates the ability of our approach to perform induction over LOD. Moreover, the approach described here could be applied to other domains covered by LOD.

The imbalance between GO-term facts and other facts in the learning dataset leads to a majority of predicates referring to GO-terms in the theories. One way to avoid the overwhelming effect of the GO-term is to limit their number on the basis of the evidence code associated with GO annotations. These codes specify the way an annotation has been assigned to a protein. Filtering out annotations with *IEA* (Inferred from Electronic Annotation) code would decrease the volume of GO annotations and restrain the study to well established ones. Another solution is to run two separate experiments on two complementary datasets composed on the one hand of GO-term facts and on the other hand, of other predicates. This would lead to two separate theories that would then be combined by designing and evaluating a global prediction model as proposed in [31, 32]. This will require a selection of the best rules from each theory. Indeed, we are currently studying methods for evaluating the statistical significance of the theory rules, *i.e.*, how specific they are to the genes responsible for intellectual disability when compared to all other known genes. Such evaluation is also a mean to assess the novelty of extracted knowledge before biological validation.

References

[1] Bizer, C., Heath, T., Berners-Lee, T.: Linked Data - The Story So Far. Int. J. Semantic Web Inf. Syst. 5(3), 1–22 (2009)

[2] Antezana, E., Kuiper, M., Mironov, V.: Biological knowledge management: the emerging role of the Semantic Web technologies. Briefings in Bioinformatics 10(4), 392–407 (2009)

[3] Belleau, F., Nolin, M.-A., Tourigny, N., Rigault, P., Morissette, J.: Bio2RDF: Towards a mashup to build bioinformatics knowledge systems. Journal of Biomedical Informatics 41(5), 706–716 (2008); Semantic Mashup of Biomedical Data

[4] Samwald, M., Jentzsch, A., Bouton, C., Kallesøe, C., Willighagen, E.L., Hajagos, J., Marshall, M.S., Prud'hommeaux, E., Hassanzadeh, O., Pichler, E., Stephens, S.: Linked open drug data for pharmaceutical research and development. J. Cheminformatics 3, 19 (2011)

[5] Kinjo, A.R., Suzuki, H., Yamashita, R., Ikegawa, Y., Kudou, T., Igarashi, R., Kengaku, Y., Cho, H., Standley, D.M., Nakagawa, A., Nakamura, H.: Protein Data Bank Japan (PDBj): maintaining a structural data archive and resource description framework format. Nucleic Acids Research 40 (Database-Issue), 453–460 (2012)

[6] The EBI RDF Platform, http://www.ebi.ac.uk/rdf/

[7] Ashburner, M., Ball, C.A., Blake, J.A., Botstein, D., Butler, H., Cherry, M., Davis, A.P., Dolinski, K., Dwight, S.S., Eppig, J.T., et al.: Gene Ontology: tool for the unification of biology. Nature Genetics 25(1), 25–29 (2000)

[8] Coulet, A., Smaïl-Tabbone, M., Benlian, P., Napoli, A., Devignes, M.-D.: Ontology-guided data preparation for discovering genotype-phenotype relationships. BMC Bioinformatics 9(suppl. 4), S3 (2008)

[9] Coulet, A., Smaïl-Tabbone, M., Napoli, A., Devignes, M.-D.: Ontology-based knowledge discovery in pharmacogenomics. In: Software Tools and Algorithms for Biological Systems, pp. 357–366. Springer (2011)

[10] Good, B.M., Wilkinson, M.D.: The Life Sciences Semantic Web is Full of Creeps!. Briefings in Bioinformatics 7(3), 275–286 (2006)

[11] Marshall, M.S., Boyce, R.D., Deus, H.F., Zhao, J., Willighagen, E.L., Samwald, M., Pichler, E., Hajagos, J., Prud'hommeaux, E., Stephens, S.: Emerging practices for mapping and linking life sciences data using RDF - A case series. J. Web Sem. 14, 2–13 (2012)

[12] Alam, M., Chekol, M.W., Coulet, A., Napoli, A., Smaïl-Tabbone, M.: Lattice Based Data Access (LBDA): An Approach for Organizing and Accessing Linked Open Data in Biology. In: Proceedings of the International Workshop on Data Mining on Linked Data, DMoLD 2013 (2013)

[13] Callahan, A., Cruz-Toledo, J., Dumontier, M.: Querying Bio2RDF Linked Open Data with a Global Schema. In: Proceedings of Bio-ontologies SIG (2012)

[14] Wilkinson, M.D., Vandervalk, B.P., McCarthy, E.L.: The Semantic Automated Discovery and Integration (SADI) Web service Design-Pattern, API and Reference Implementation. J. Biomedical Semantics 2, 8 (2011)

[15] Lopes, P., Oliveira, J.L.: COEUS: "semantic web in a box" for biomedical applications. J. Biomedical Semantics 3, 11 (2012)

[16] Gangemi, A., Nuzzolese, A.G., Presutti, V., Draicchio, F., Musetti, A., Ciancarini, P.: Automatic typing of dBpedia entities. In: Cudré-Mauroux, P., Heflin, J., Sirin, E., Tudorache, T., Euzenat, J., Hauswirth, M., Parreira, J.X., Hendler, J., Schreiber, G., Bernstein, A., Blomqvist, E. (eds.) ISWC 2012, Part I. LNCS, vol. 7649, pp. 65–81. Springer, Heidelberg (2012)

[17] Ngonga Ngomo, A.-C.: Link discovery with guaranteed reduction ratio in affine spaces with minkowski measures. In: Cudré-Mauroux, P., Heflin, J., Sirin, E., Tudorache, T., Euzenat, J., Hauswirth, M., Parreira, J.X., Hendler, J., Schreiber, G., Bernstein, A., Blomqvist, E. (eds.) ISWC 2012, Part I. LNCS, vol. 7649, pp. 378–393. Springer, Heidelberg (2012)

[18] Xu, M., Wang, Z., Bie, R., Li, J., Zheng, C., Ke, W., Zhou, M.: Discovering Missing Semantic Relations between Entities in Wikipedia. In: Alani, H., Kagal, L., Fokoue, A., Groth, P., Biemann, C., Parreira, J.X., Aroyo, L., Noy, N., Welty, C., Janowicz, K. (eds.) ISWC 2013, Part I. LNCS, vol. 8218, pp. 673–686. Springer, Heidelberg (2013)

[19] Brenninkmeijer, C.Y.A., Dunlop, I., Goble, C.A., Gray, A.J.G., Pettifer, S., Stevens, R.: Computing Identity Co-Reference Across Drug Discovery Datasets. In: Proceedings of the 6th International Workshop on Semantic Web Applications and Tools for Life Sciences, SWAT4LS 2013 (2013)

[20] Percha, B., Garten, Y., Altman, R.B.: Discovery and explanation of drug-drug interactions via text mining. In: Pacific Symposium on Biocomputing. Pacific Symposium on Biocomputing, pp. 410–421. World Scientific (2012)

[21] Pathak, J., Kiefer, R.C., Chute, C.G.: Mining Anti-coagulant Drug-Drug Interactions from Electronic Health Records Using Linked Data. In: Baker, C.J.O., Butler, G., Jurisica, I. (eds.) DILS 2013. LNCS, vol. 7970, pp. 128–140. Springer, Heidelberg (2013)

[22] d'Aquin, M., Kronberger, G., Suárez-Figueroa, M.C.: Combining data mining and ontology engineering to enrich ontologies and linked data. In: Workshop: Knowledge Discovery and Data Mining Meets Linked Open Data-Know@ LOD at Extended Semantic Web Conference (ESWC), vol. 2012 (2012)

[23] Galárraga, L.A., Teflioudi, C., Hose, K., Suchanek, F.: Amie: association rule mining under incomplete evidence in ontological knowledge bases. In: Proceedings of the 22nd International Conference on World Wide Web, pp. 413–422. International World Wide Web Conferences Steering Committee (2013)

[24] Muggleton, S.: Inductive Logic Programming. New Generation Computing 8(4), 295–318 (1991)

[25] Muggleton, S., De Raedt, L.: Inductive logic programming: Theory and methods. The Journal of Logic Programming 19(20), 629–679 (1994)

[26] Srinivasan, A.: The Aleph Manual (2007), http://www.comlab.ox.ac.uk/oucl/research/areas/machlearn/Aleph/

[27] Inlow, J.K., Restifo, L.L.: Molecular and comparative genetics of mental retarda-
tion. Genetics 166(2), 835–881 (2004)

[28] Berthold, M.R., Cebron, N., Dill, F., Gabriel, T.R., Kötter, T., Meinl, T., Ohl,
P., Thiel, K., Wiswedel, B.: KNIME-the Konstanz information miner: version 2.0
and beyond. ACM SIGKDD Explorations Newsletter 11(1), 26–31 (2009)

[29] Grisoni, R., Bresso, E., Devignes, M.-D., Smaïl-Tabbone, M.: Méthodologie et
outils pour l'extraction de connaissances par Programmation Logique Inductive
(PLI) (Poster). In: 13 ème Conférence Francophone sur l'Extraction et la Gestion
des Connaissances- EGC 2013, Toulouse, France (2013)

[30] van Karnebeek, C.D., Stockler, S.: Treatable inborn errors of metabolism caus-
ing intellectual disability: a systematic literature review. Molecular Genetics and
Metabolism 105(3), 368–381 (2012)

[31] Berthold, M.R., Morik, K., Siebes, A.: Parallel Universes and Local Patterns.
Dagstuhl Seminar Proceedings, vol. 07181 (2007)

[32] Knobbe, A., Crémilleux, B., Fürnkranz, J., Scholz, M.: From Local Patterns to
Global Models: The LeGo Approach to Data Mining. In: International Work-
shop From Local Patterns to Global Models co-located with ECML/PKDD 2008,
Antwerp, Belgium, pp. 1–16 (September 2008)

Data Integration between Swedish National Clinical Health Registries and Biobanks Using an Availability System

Ola Spjuth[1], Jani Heikkinen[2,3], Jan-Eric Litton[1],
Juni Palmgren[1,3], and Maria Krestyaninova[2,3,4]

[1] Department of Medical Epidemiology and Biostatistics
and Swedish e-Science Research Center,
Karolinska Institutet, P.O. Box 281, SE-171 77 Stockholm, Sweden
[2] Uniquer Sarl, 12 rue de la Mercerie, 1003, Lausanne, Switzerland
[3] Institute for Molecular Medicine Finland FIMM, University of Helsinki, Helsinki,
FI-00290, Finland
[4] Eawag, Überlandstrasse 133, P.O. Box 611, 8600 Dübendorf, Switzerland
{ola.spjuth,jan-eric.litton,juni.palmgren}@ki.se,
{jani,masha}@simbioms.org

Abstract. Linking biobank data, such as molecular profiles, with clinical phenotypes is of great importance in epidemiological and predictive studies. A comprehensive overview of various data sources that can be combined in order to power up a study is a key factor in the design. Clinical data stored in health registries and biobank data in research projects are commonly provisioned in different database systems and governed by separate organizations, making the integration process challenging and hampering biomedical investigations. We here describe the integration of data on prostate cancer from a clinical health registry with data from a biobank, and its provisioning in the SAIL availability system. We demonstrate the implications of using the actual raw data, data transformed to availability data, and availability data which has been subjected to anonymization techniques to reduce the risk of re-identification. Our results show that an availability system such as SAIL with integrated clinical and biobank data can be a valuable tool for planning new studies and finding interesting subsets to investigate further. We also show that an availability system can deliver useful insights even when the data has been subjected to anonymization techniques.

Keywords: Data integration, health registry, biobanks, availability system, anonymization.

1 Introduction

Health registries containing information on patients, diseases, and treatments are important for ensuring high quality in health care but are also gold mines for medical and epidemiological research [1]. With the advent of new technology to measure biomarkers, studies in molecular epidemiology have become increasingly

H. Galhardas and E. Rahm (Eds.): DILS 2014, LNBI 8574, pp. 32–40, 2014.

more common and biobanks have emerged to store biological samples such as blood, plasma and urine as well as record data from their analysis [2]. As a result, there has been a growing demand to connect information in health registries with molecular data in biobanks for example to seek insights into underlying reasons of diseases or to improve predictions [3].

Sweden has a big advantage with a multitude of national databases, allowing to explore e,g, how genes and the environment influence disease [4]. The country's national health care system gives each person an identification number at birth (PID) and maintains health records in registries. While health registries in many cases have been around for several years and are governed by the health care, biobanks are recent phenomena and often form part of relatively new research infrastructures. The difference in governing organizations is an obstacle when aiming to combine data sources, due to differences in the underlying requirements and data reporting standards [5]. Furthermore the actual content is sensitive and hence there are also issues with security and privacy restrictions which also vary from organization to organization [6]. The many challenges of integrating biomedical data are nicely summarized by Harris et al.[7]

Linking data between registries and biobanks is in most cases done via personal identifiers, which can be pseudonymized to reduce the chance of re-identification. However, if gaining access to the data it can still be possible in some cases to identify individuals using prior information [8]. For example it has been shown that it is possible to resolve an individual in a collection with only a fraction of their DNA made available [9,10]. Methods for statistical disclosure control (SDC) are aimed at protecting the confidentiality of individuals and involves modifying data so that the risk of re-identification of individuals is reduced to an acceptable level. This might include suppressing (removing) information, generalizing, or perturbing values. A commonly used method is k-anonymity [11,12] where attributes are suppressed or generalized until each row is identical with at least k-1 other rows. At this point the data is said to be k-anonymous. Of importance for disclosure control methods is to seek an optimal balance between the improvement in confidentiality protection and the reduction in data quality. SDC has been successfully applied in several bioscience projects, such as Jerboa [13] and DataSHIELD [14].

Data availability systems take a pragmatic approach for linking data by operating on metadata level; information is provided for each entity regarding whether a value for a given metadata term (can be a phenotype for instance) exists or not. The value per se is not disclosed, hence many privacy issues are avoided [15]. In other words, an availability system would give a rather accurate estimate of how much relevant data is available at which location, based on the prior agreement on the metadata definitions between the data providers and data analysts. Availability systems have previously been implemented in large-scale genetic studies but primarily been focused on integrating data from multiple biobanks [16]. The aim of such setups has mainly been to allow researchers to explore if larger sample sizes can be achieved by combining data from two or more biobanks.

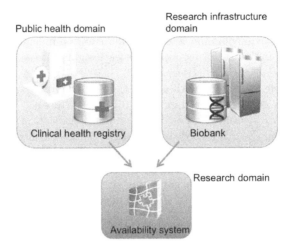

Fig. 1. We show how an availability system can be used to integrate data from clinical health registries with biobanks. The different domains of health care, research infrastructure, and general research makes this process challenging due to legal, political, semantic, and privacy issues.

In this manuscript we show how availability systems can be used to integrate data from a clinical health registry with data from a biobank (Fig. 1). We also describe how SDC methods can be applied to strengthen privacy preservation in such settings, and exemplify with three different scenarios with varying privacy levels for the same data and detail their implications for querying and results.

2   Methods

2.1   Data

We used health registry data from the Swedish national prostate cancer quality registry comprising information on diagnosis, treatment, and follow-up in prostate cancer treatment. The data was delivered as a CSV file. We used biobank data from the Karolinska Institutet, Sweden, containing data on biospecimens in the form of DNA, Serum, and Blood from patients. This data was also delivered as a CSV file. The variables in the datasets can be seen in Table 1. Both registry and biobank data contained personal identifiers (PID) in the form of Swedish personal number, allowing data to be linked using these.

Since the data used in this project is subject to privacy regulations it is not possible to provide an open system with public access. For demonstration purposes we simulated 1000 patients with prostate cancer with the biobank metadata terms as the health registry. We also simulated 1000 samples with the biobank metadata terms and ensured a substantial overlap between the collections as linked by PIDs (Table 2). While the simulation method was based on a

Table 1. Variables in the health registry and biobank datasets. The personal identifier (PID) allows for linking records.

Prostate cancer registry

Name	Description
PID	Unique identifier for the patient
AGE	Age of patient
YEAR_DIAG	Year of diagnosis
LKF_VALUE	Structured location in Sweden where patient lived
PSA	Prostate-specific antigen (a biomarker for prostate cancer) [17], value at time of diagnosis
Gleason	Gleason grade [18] at time of diagnosis
T_STAGE	Size of the original (primary) tumor and whether it has invaded nearby tissue [19]
N_STAGE	Involvement of nearby (regional) lymph nodes [19]
M_STAGE	Indication of distant metastasis [19]

Biobank

Name	Description
PID	Unique identifier for the patient
DNA	1 if DNA is stored for sample
PLASMA	1 if plasma is stored for sample
SAMPLING_YEAR	Year the sample was obtained
QUESTIONNAIRE	1 if patient has answered a questionnaire on lifestyle

rather simple univariate method, the resulting data was sufficient for demonstration purposes and could be put on the web with public access. From the simulated data we then constructed three subsets: A) Actual values for the health registry and availability data for the biobank, B) availability values for the health registry and the the biobank, C) anonymized availability values for the health registry and the the biobank. The simulated data is hence on the same structure as the original data, but the values do not originate from real patients.

2.2   Data Availability System

We chose the SAIL data availability system, originally developed for integrating data from biobanks [15] and used in the SUMMIT [http://www.imi-summit.eu/] and ENGAGE [http://www.euengage.org/] consortia [16]. SAIL operates on metadata level and provides an interface for harmonisation and submission of sample and phenotype information, as well as a graphical user interface when users can construct queries and create reports quantifying the data available at various sources for a given set of metadata terms [20]. SAIL was chosen as it is open source and allows for resource discovery across data archives at the level of individual records, which is not readily available in other solutions.

Table 2. Schematic presentation of the merged dataset of 1000 patients from the health registry with 1000 biospecimens from the biobank. Highlighted area shows a subset of individuals for whom records are present both in the biobank and in the registry.

PID	DNA	PLASMA	SAMPL_YEAR	QUEST	LKF_VALUE	YEAR_DIAG	T_STAGE
1	d1	pl1	SY1	q1			
2	d2	pl2	SY2	q2			
3	d3	pl3	SY3	q3	LKF3	YD3	T3
4	d4	pl4	SY4	q4	LKF4	YD4	T4
5					LKF5	YD5	T5
6					LKF6	YD6	T6

2.3 Anonymization Procedure

We applied a k-anonymization algorithm implemented in the R-package sdcMicro [21] to suppress the AGE and LKF columns and hence reduce the risk of re-identification. We used k=10 and this suppressed 75 AGE entries but no LKF entries. Having k=10 ensures that no group of patients with a certain value will be of 9 or less individuals. The LKF, describing the location in Sweden, turned out to already satisfy this condition and hence no entries were suppressed.

3 Results and Discussion

We set up three SAIL instances, one for each of the three datasets, providing different views on the original integrated simulated data with implications on data expressiveness, sensitivity, but also querying capability. Instance A with

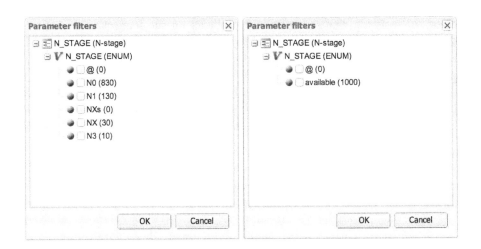

Fig. 2. Querying capability for the parameter N-stage in the original data in instance A (left) and the availability data in instance B (right)

actual values for the health registry and availability data for the biobank provides full access to querying and data. Instance B has some variables transformed into availability type (1 or 0) which limits queries to return results on the form if data exists or not, for example it is not possible to query on different N-stages but rather on the form if there is N-stage information available (Fig 2). Instance C contained the data that also was subjected for anonymization, which was set up in order to demonstrate the implications for an availability system with respect to details in querying and results.

In order to construct the three SAIL instances we have created one set of metadata terms that encompasses all those characteristics for biospecimen in biobank and in registry that were to be used for filtering (age, cancer stage, DNA availability, etc). Once a common format was established, we used it as a configuration for the SAIL system, i.e. created what is called vocabulary, which is a set of standardized terms for each of which sample records can be linked and thus when filtering a number of samples available for a chosen set of terms can be calculated. For clarity purposes it should be noted here that the SAIL system by the way of its design consists of two parts: a) semantic information: metadata terms, information about the them and relatedness between; and b) biospecimen collection per se: patient record or sample id, collection it came from etc. For the purpose of the feasibility study that we present here, a set of metadata terms were selected from a complete set of variables used by the Swedish Cancer Centre [22] and from the variables recorded at the biobank. Upon completion of the metadata definition and configuration of the SAIL system, the three SAIL instances were populated with data. URLs to the instances are available on the supporting web page[1]. The three instances allowed us to explore how much information in fact is needed by analytics in order to make effective decisions about study design.

In order to illustrate what we mean by different depth of information that can constitute the content of an availability system, let us first consider the following query: *"Select all patients in the age span 70 to 80 years which have a Gleason score recorded in the quality registry and which have blood plasma stored in the biobank"*. The overlap between the three sets of records is 45, meaning that out of total number of 1500 individual records, 45 satisfy the criteria and records and biospecimen for whom can be located in the registry and the biobank (Figure 3).

Let us now compare how different the results are with the same filters but in the case of anonymized data. Table 3 presents the results of such query run on two different instances of the availability system: populated with availability data (B) and populated with anonymized availability data (C). This shows that the anonymization has suppressed a number of patients which we now are unable to identify with the query. This is the price we pay for reducing the risk of re-identification.

Note that an availability system can be set up at several locations with different views on the same data, such as on Internet with public access or on an intranet with restricted access. The main goal of the materials that we have

---

[1] www.ecpc.e-science.se/applications/data-availability

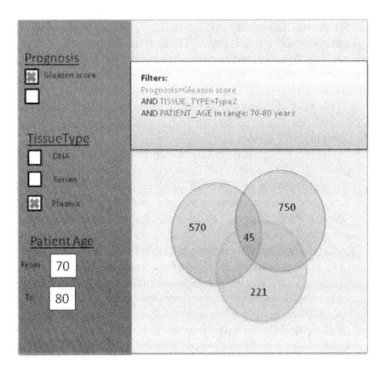

Fig. 3. Conceptual view of filtering a merged dataset by the biobank and quality registry variables Prognosis and age are variables recorded at the registry, while tissue type information comes from the biobank. In this query, the blue circle corresponds to the query result 'Prognosis=Gleason score' with 570 matching patients, the red circle 'Tissue_Type=Type2' with 750 matching patients and green circle 'Patient-AGE in range 70-80 years' with 221 matches. The intersection satisfying all three queries is 45 patients. The total number of patients is 1532, and there are indeed some patients that do not fit any of the three search criteria.

presented here is to share practical experience of integrating biomedical data that come from two very different sources and to provide guidance and suggestion for practices in the future:

1) How much time and effort to be invested into creation of a common set of metadata is to be weighed against how well the scope of the research studies is defined; a graphical user interface allowing to create variables in a collegial fashion (in consultation between experts) is an essential enhancer of the cross-data source integration, e.g. registry data with biobank data.

2) Instead of trying to reach one-for-all resolution on the privacy and security restrictions create a range of instances of the same system with the same metadata and let the stakeholders decide how much clinical, biological and medical data can be available for querying under various security and anoymization settings.

Table 3. Results for the query All patients in the age span 70 to 80 years which has a Gleason score recorded and blood plasma stored in the biobank. Lower numbers in the Result column for dataset C is due to suppressed data in the anonymization and is the price to pay for reducing the risk of re-identification.

Instance	Records	AGE	Gleason	Plasma	Result
B (availability)	1532	221	570	750	43
C (anonymized availability)	1532	190	569	750	37

4 Conclusions

We have demonstrated in this manuscript how data from biobanks and health registries can be interlinked using availability systems. We have also considered a complementary approach of preprocessing raw data into availability data or into anonymized availability data which implies a trade-off between data security and risk of re-identification against flexibility in queries and precision of results. Being able to quantify e.g. re-identification risks can allow authorities and regulators to establish guidelines and best-practices for data publication, and we envision that availability system with anonymized data will play an important role in biomedical informatics in the future.

References

1. Solomon, D.J., Henry, R.C., Hogan, J.G., Van Amburg, G.H., Taylor, J.: Evaluation and implementation of public health registries. Public Health Rep. 106(2), 142–150 (1991)
2. McCarthy, M.I., Abecasis, G.R., Cardon, L.R., Goldstein, D.B., Little, J., Ioannidis, J.P.A., Hirschhorn, J.N.: Genome-wide association studies for complex traits: consensus, uncertainty and challenges. Nat. Rev. Genet. 9(5), 356–369 (2008)
3. Manolio, T.A.: Genomewide association studies and assessment of the risk of disease. N. Engl. J. Med. 363(2), 166–176 (2010)
4. Kaiser, J.: Swedish bioscience. working sweden's population gold mine. Science 293(5539), 2375 (2001)
5. Fortier, I., Doiron, D., Little, J., Ferretti, V., L'Heureux, F., Stolk, R.P., Knoppers, B.M., Hudson, T.J., Burton, P.R.: Is rigorous retrospective harmonization possible? application of the datashaper approach across 53 large studies. Int. J. Epidemiol. 40(5), 1314–1328 (2011)
6. Reiter, J.P., Kinney, S.K.: Sharing confidential data for research purposes: a primer. Epidemiology 22(5), 632–635 (2011)
7. Harris, J.R., Burton, P., Knoppers, B.M., Lindpaintner, K., Bledsoe, M., Brookes, A.J., Budin-Ljøsne, I., Chisholm, R., Cox, D., Deschênes, M., Fortier, I., Hainaut, P., Hewitt, R., Kaye, J., Litton, J.E., Metspalu, A., Ollier, B., Palmer, L.J., Palotie, A., Pasterk, M., Perola, M., Riegman, P.H.J., van Ommen, G.J., Yuille, M., Zatloukal, K.: Toward a roadmap in global biobanking for health. Eur. J. Hum. Genet. 20(11), 1105–1111 (2012)
8. Dankar, F.K., El Emam, K., Neisa, A., Roffey, T.: Estimating the re-identification risk of clinical data sets. BMC Med. Inform. Decis. Mak. 12, 66 (2012)

9. Homer, N., Szelinger, S., Redman, M., Duggan, D., Tembe, W., Muehling, J., Pearson, J.V., Stephan, D.A., Nelson, S.F., Craig, D.W.: Resolving individuals contributing trace amounts of dna to highly complex mixtures using high-density snp genotyping microarrays. PLoS Genet. 4(8), e1000167 (2008)
10. Gymrek, M., McGuire, A.L., Golan, D., Halperin, E., Erlich, Y.: Identifying personal genomes by surname inference. Science 339(6117), 321–324 (2013)
11. El Emam, K., Dankar, F.K.: Protecting privacy using k-anonymity. Journal of the American Medical Informatics Association 15, 627–637 (2008)
12. Samarati, P., Sweeney, L.: Protecting privacy when disclosing information: k-anonymity and its enforcement through generalization and suppression. Technical report (1998)
13. Avillach, P., Coloma, P.M., Gini, R., Schuemie, M., Mougin, F., Dufour, J.C., Mazzaglia, G., Giaquinto, C., Fornari, C., Herings, R., Molokhia, M., Pedersen, L., Fourrier-Réglat, A., Fieschi, M., Sturkenboom, M., van der Lei, J., Pariente, A., Trifirò, G.: EU-ADR consortium: Harmonization process for the identification of medical events in eight european healthcare databases: the experience from the eu-adr project. J. Am. Med. Inform. Assoc. 20(1), 184–192 (2013)
14. Wolfson, M., Wallace, S.E., Masca, N., Rowe, G., Sheehan, N.A., Ferretti, V., LaFlamme, P., Tobin, M.D., Macleod, J., Little, J., Fortier, I., Knoppers, B.M., Burton, P.R.: Datashield: resolving a conflict in contemporary bioscience–performing a pooled analysis of individual-level data without sharing the data. Int. J. Epidemiol. 39(5), 1372–1382 (2010)
15. Gostev, M., Fernandez-Banet, J., Rung, J., Dietrich, J., Prokopenko, I., Ripatti, S., McCarthy, M.I., Brazma, A., Krestyaninova, M.: Sail–a software system for sample and phenotype availability across biobanks and cohorts. Bioinformatics 27(4), 589–591 (2011)
16. ENGAGE Consortium: Data sharing in large research consortia: experiences and recommendations from engage. Eur. J. Hum. Genet. 22(3), 317–321 (2014)
17. Kuriyama, M., Wang, M.C., Papsidero, L.D., Killian, C.S., Shimano, T., Valenzuela, L., Nishiura, T., Murphy, G.P., Chu, T.M.: Quantitation of prostate-specific antigen in serum by a sensitive enzyme immunoassay. Cancer Research 40(12), 4658–4662 (1980)
18. Milette, F., Larivière, L., Piché, J.: Gleason grading of prostatic biopsies. Am. J. Surg. Pathol. 24(10),1443–1444 (2000)
19. NCI: Cancer staging, http://www.cancer.gov/cancertopics/factsheet/detection/
20. SIMBIOMS: Sail user guide, http://www.simbioms.org/wordpress/wp-content/uploads/2013/08/SAIL_documentation.pdf
21. Templ, M.: scdMicro: A package for statistical disclosure control in R. ISI (2007)
22. Swedish Cancer Centre: Variable description for the prostate cancer quality regsitry, http://www.cancercentrum.se/Global/Diagnoser/prostatacancer/Prostata_variabelbeskr_130101.pdf

Data Management Experiences and Best Practices from the Perspective of a Plant Research Institute

Daniel Arend*, Christian Colmsee, Helmut Knüpffer, Markus Oppermann,
Uwe Scholz, Danuta Schüler, Stephan Weise, and Matthias Lange

Leibniz Institute of Plant Genetics and Crop Plant Research (IPK), OT Gatersleben,
Corrensstr. 3, 06446 Stadt Seeland, Germany
`arendd@ipk-gatersleben.de`

Abstract. Research in life sciences faces increasing amounts of cross-domain data, also kown as "big data". This has notable effects on IT-departments and the dry lab desk alike. In this paper, we report on experiences from a decade of data management in a plant research institute. We explain the switch from personally managed files and heterogeneous information systems towards a centrally organised storage management. In particular, we discuss lessons that were learned within the last decade of productive research, data generation and software development from the perspective of a modern plant research institute and present the results of a strategic realignment of the data management infrastructure. Finally, we summarise the challenges which were solved and the questions which are still open.

1 Challenges in the Management of Research Data

The "big data" challenge has reached the life science community [10,12] and necessitates a sustainable infrastructure for storing, exchanging and publishing research data. The Leibniz Institute of Plant Genetics and Crop Plant Research (IPK) is committed to the conservation and valorisation of plant genetic resources. Its research agenda comprises upstream and downstream analyses in the fields of genetics, physiology and cell biology aiming at a broad understanding of plants at molecular, cellular and organismic levels. The IPK maintains the German Federal *ex situ* Genebank of Agricultural and Horticultural Crop Species, which represents the largest collection of its kind in Western Europe, totalling over 150,000 living accessions of crop plants and their wild relatives, predominantly as seeds. It has been continuously developed over the past 70 years and provides the basis for follow-up research. Crop plants are important for the human nutrition. The worldwide food production faces problems like climate change or limited water resources. However, it is necessary to increase the food production by 70% to 100% by 2050 to keep pace with the predicted

---

* Corresponding author.

H. Galhardas and E. Rahm (Eds.): DILS 2014, LNBI 8574, pp. 41–49, 2014.

population growth and changes in diet. At the IPK, about 30 research groups are conducting research as well as managing the research data. This data comprises mass spectroscopy data giving information about the metabolite content of plants, Next Generation Sequencing (NGS) data providing insights into the genotype, and high-throughput phenotyping data, amongst others.

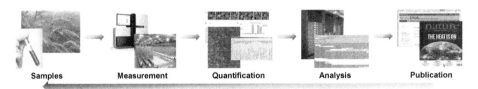

Fig. 1. General pipeline from experiment to publication

Figure 1 shows a simplified illustration of the research data lifecycle such as might be found anywhere around the world. After an overview about the historically evolved research data management, we give recommendations from a practical point of view. The arising infrastructural changes are discussed subsequently and summarised as an experience report.

1.1 File Management

Currently, the IPK's IT stores more than 80 million files on a hierarchical storage management (HSM) system with a data volume of more than 200 terabytes. In consequence, data management is a major task in the daily research process, but by far the least attractive one. Figure 2 shows the distribution of the data files and their volume.

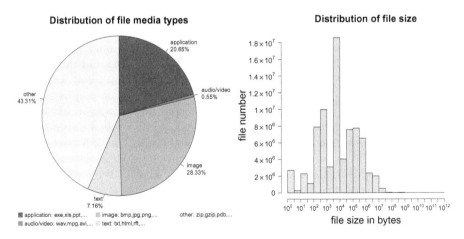

Fig. 2. Properties of HSM managed files: In January 2014, the HSM managed 231TB data in 80 million single files of 3,185 different file types. Their distribution over 5 major MIME media types is shown in the left chart. The distribution of file sizes is shown in the right chart, the largest single file size being 610GB.

1.2   Databases and Information Systems

Before the first IPK bioinformatics IT infrastructure was established at the turn of the millennium, plant-specific data was managed in heterogeneous formats by individual research groups, using various storage systems. In subsequent years, a strategy for data integration was developed as the fundament for cross-domain analysis of plant biological data [7].

In order to support the great diversity of research fields at the IPK, a variety of information systems and tools was developed over the years. Table 1 shows a representative sample of developments. The complete list can be found at *http://bioinformatics.ipk-gatersleben.de*. These systems form a valuable resource for cross-domain data integration and analysis. However several challenges remain with a decentralised data storage approach within one institute. The most critical drawback is that every application uses its own database schema and/or storage backend. Consequently, new projects usually tend to new independent developments. Considering the maintenance effort, it appears doubtful whether such a strategy would prove successful over the long term. In contrast, a life science research institute like the IPK would strongly benefit from a central IT-infrastructure dealing with all aspects of data management, including data storage, data retrieval and data publication.

2   A Practitioner's View on Life Science Data Management

In 2010, the IPK conducted a study to analyse the requirements for an institute-wide information system and to evaluate approaches, i.e. a Laboratory Information and Management System (LIMS). Different research groups were interviewed and their daily labour processes were analysed. Thereby, general requirements for a sustainable data management could be found (Fig. 3). Besides functional needs, there are also several technical and infrastructural demands that have to be met.

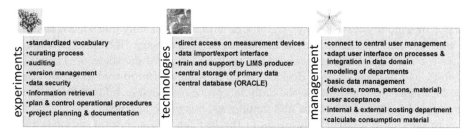

Fig. 3. Cut-out of IPK's requirement analysis for data management & lab documentation.

A fundamental problem is the lack of a standardised vocabulary for the documentation of experiments and lab processes. This lack makes it difficult to reuse or search specific data, and it complicates documentation. Furthermore, since

Table 1. Representative sample of information systems and tools developed in-house, sorted from genetic(1) to phenotypic(6) level

---

1 - **CR-EST:** http://pgrc.ipk-gatersleben.de/cr-est
The IPK **Crop EST Database** (CR-EST) [8] contains data about Expressed Sequence Tags of barley, wheat, pea, potato, petunia and tobacco as well as information about cDNA libraries, DNA sequences, assembly and annotation.

2 - **OPTIMAS-DW:** http://www.optimas-bioenergy.org/optimas_dw
OPTIMAS-DW [2] is a comprehensive data warehouse for maize allowing storage and retrieval of experimental data from multiple -omics domains. It supports systems biologists by providing data from transcriptomics to phenomics level.

3 - **MetaCrop:** http://metacrop.ipk-gatersleben.de
The **MetaCrop** information system [11] contains fine-grained data (down to compartment level) about metabolic pathways of several major crop plant species, including kinetic information. In order to ensure a high data quality, all information was curated manually from the literature.

4 - **GBIS/I:** http://gbis.ipk-gatersleben.de
The **Genebank Information System** (GBIS) is the central database-driven information system for managing the accessions of the IPK genebank. Its externally visible component GBIS/I enables public users to access information about them and to order seed samples.

5 - **GSCC:** http://www.ipk-gatersleben.de/databases/gscc
The **Garlic and Shallot Core Collection** (GSCC) [3] contains images on the outside view of plants, bulbs and cloves, bulb structure, field cultivation, inflorescence and bulbils etc., passport and characterisation data, genotype classification, and image sequences on the ontogenesis of selected accessions.

6 - **Mansfeld-DB:** http://mansfeld.ipk-gatersleben.de
Mansfeld's World Database of Agricultural and Horticultural Crops [6] comprises information on the taxonomy, cultivation regions, domestication, uses etc. on ca. 6,100 species of agricultural and horticultural cultivated plants.

---

each research group has its own data management approach using CDs, USB drives or a cloud-based storage, the risk of data loss is usually quite high. Hence, a uniform and sustainable data management is necessary. Technical prerequisites for such a solution already exist, such as a central database or a reliable storage and backup system. Besides the large volume of produced data, also basic information important for the daily lab processes, such as information about available hardware, chemicals and employees, has to be handled.

Considering infrastructural needs in the last few years, several national and international organisations analysed the common research process [5,13], such as nestor [9] or the DataCite consortium [4]. They also provide suggestions for a good scientific practice to guarantee a long-term usability of digital objects. Consequently, a homogeneous storage system is necessary, which complies with physical and software requirements as well as with organisational demands (Tab. 2).

Table 2. Hardware, software & organisational requirements for a long-term archive

Storage requirements	Software demands	Organisational requirements
• Redundant data storage • Diverse storage media • Standard storage devices • Frequent data migration	• Long-term readability • Format migration • Format/environment emulation	• Permanent staff • Mixed core and project funding • Central hardware procurement process and project coordination

2.1 The Pros and Cons of LIMS Based Data Management

The IPK LIMS, introduced in 2011, has many advantages and provides a broad functionality, but there are still shortcomings and open issues. Having evolved over time and been adjusted to special requirements, there are several other information systems existing beside the LIMS (see Tab. 1). The systems are co-existing, some of them having mutual access to some data, but in general the connection between them is still an open task.

Although the use of the different LIMS modules is very comfortable for the various research groups, extensive training is necessary. End users have different levels of computational skills and strong personal preferences concerning data handling. Thus, it is challenging to convince users that using the central LIMS offers major advantages in the long run. Therefore, it is important to involve the users already in the process of the development, but, needless to say, this can be very time-consuming. Here, providing a group- or even institute-wide policy can help to define rules about how to handle data. Furthermore, it can be a problem that the LIMS does not have an out-of-the-box module for making stored data accessible to public users, e.g., via a web interface as in the case of the systems described in section 1.2. Its clear advantage is the homogeneous use of the central storage backend.

2.2 Consistent Data Publication

Another major task is to make data long-term citable. Many data resources are too large or have no acceptable representation to put them directly into a publication, i.e. a journal article. Usually, authors refer to external resources using different solutions; e.g., the data can be uploaded to public, domain specific long-term archives, such as the Sequence Read Archive for NGS raw data or the BioModels database for modeling results. Many archives need specific metadata and provide different ways to upload the data. Thus, if permitted by the publishing journal, it is usually faster to transfer the datasets to publicly available web servers hosted by the authors' institutes and adding the URLs to the "materials" sections of the respective articles. In reality, after only a short time this often leads to dead links, because resources for maintenance are lacking.

Since 2010, the IPK is registered as a data centre in the DataCite consortium, which provides an alternative solution by using the persistent Digital Object Identifier (DOI). The DataCite resolving service guarantees the long-term availability. By now, DOIs are not only used in life sciences, but also in social sciences, bibliography, and other fields. However, in the last years we realised that the interest in registering DOIs at the IPK was not very pronounced. Thus, we started the development of the e!DAL-API [1] as a general software framework for data storage and publication in order to increase the usage of this service.

3   Lessons Learned: Strategic Realignment of IPK's Research Data Management

Handling research data is an important task in IPK's research strategy and particularly a central component along the value-added chain towards scientific publications, patents and biotechnological innovations. Furthermore, it is an economical asset on a national and international level, which needs to be preserved.

These considerations and the experiences from a decade of research data management at the IPK were broadly discussed at management, scientific and administration levels. On the one hand, it can be difficult to convince researchers to follow standardised workflows and policies. On the other hand, uncontrolled and individual data management can pose a high risk of losing valuable research data. As a result, there was the conviction that it is essential to implement an intuitive and seamless data storage and documentation infrastructure, which can be easily embedded into existing workflows and will be highly accepted by scientists. Thus, a decision was made by the board of directors, which reflected the need to find compromise solutions for a sustainable research data management. The result was a plan for organisational and infrastructure actions (Tab. 3). The key actions for a realignment of IPK's data storage strategy were the establishment of core-financed permanent positions for data management, the introduction of a

Table 3. Strategic realignment of IPK's data management infrastructure

Organisational actions
1. Fusion of IT-service and scientific groups into a central bioinformatics service group with a scientific administration
2. Financing of positions from both research funds and institutional budget
3. Core-financed service team for lab data management
4. Inter-departmental coordination of bioinformatics research

Infrastructure actions
1. Centrally maintained storage systems and databases as institution-wide services:
   • Network attached storage (NetApp NAS) for project-specific data
   • Hierarchical storage management (ORACLE SAM-QFS) for archiving primary data
   • Relational database management system (ORACLE DBMS) for information systems
   • Central FTP, HTTP and application servers to support proprietary data sharing
2. Combination of in-house and public data publications system (section 1.2):
   • In-house developed information systems mainly using ORACLE APEX
   • Participation in DataCite data publication infrastructure to provide citable DOIs for FTP and HTTP shared data
   • Central service to submit data to public repositories

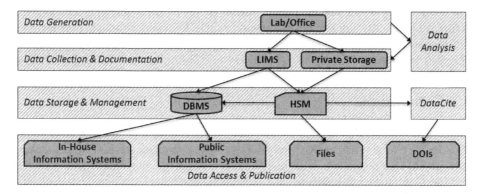

Fig. 4. IPK's emerging realignment of research data infrastructure. In this architecture, data is either generated by lab experiments, analysis software or manually maintained documentation. Self-managed files can be stored at the central NAS file server, measurement values or even binary files can be stored in the LIMS. Binary files will be uploaded transparently to the HSM system, whereas fine-grained values and metadata are stored in the central database system. Data publication can be performed by downloadable data files or information systems. In-house information systems can directly access LIMS-managed information via the central database system. Data files are accessible by a URL or a DOI, as it is recommended for stable and metadata-aware citation. Finally, data can also be uploaded to public information systems.

bioinformatics coordination, a mix of in-house technical staff and external service providers for the systems operation as well as the use of commercial storage and lab information management systems for a centrally managed service. Besides project-funded staff, permanent positions are indispensable to preserve knowhow. Thus, data can remain accessible and software tools can be maintained over a long period of time.

Another important aspect is the turning away from proprietary or open-source software for data management and information systems in favour of commercial products. The main reason is the availability of long-term support for commercial software. In case of short-term funded open-source software, there is often the problem of unsolved bugs, undocumented behaviour or simply a developer, who is losing interest in maintaining the software. Thus, the IPK focuses on a declarative (4th generation) programming platform, i.e. Oracle Application Express, in order to increase the productivity and maintainability of in-house developed information systems. Finally, the implementation of a central management system for lab processes and research data instead of dozens of individual project databases is another key to a sustainable data management infrastructure, thus enabling homogeneous and consistently annotated data and analysis results. Therefore, its integration as a central element into a data and IT infrastructure is a prerequisite for a consistent data documentation and preservation at all levels of the data-associated value-added chain. A combination of policies, reliable service and contact persons can help to convince end users of the benefits and increased efficiency for data management and publication.

Fig. 4 shows a schematic representation of IPK's data management infrastructure currently under development, which is a compromise between a self-managed, proprietary data storage and a consistently documented data management process.

4   Conclusions

In the last decade, the volume of scientific research data increased significantly, thus leading to a growing need for effective data management and information systems. In this paper, we described the evolution of the data management in a leading plant research institute. We illustrated challenges that could be solved as well as issues still open. The presentation of IPK's point of view aims at giving arguments and recommendations for a service-oriented data management in research institutes. A major conclusion is to focus on sustainable solutions, with a homogeneous but very flexible data management system in the centre. Especially at an institute with such wide-spread research topics, resulting in large volumes of multi-domain data, it is indispensable to be able to promptly react to changing requirements and new types of data.

References

1. Arend, D., Lange, M., Colmsee, C., Flemming, S., Chen, J., Scholz, U.: The e!DAL JAVA-API: Store, Share and Cite Primary Data in Life Sciences. In: IEEE International Conference on Bioinformatics and Biomedicine (BIBM), Philadelphia, U.S.A., October 4-7, pp. 511–515 (2012)
2. Colmsee, C., Mascher, M., Czauderna, T., Hartmann, A., Schlüter, U., Zellerhoff, N., Schmitz, J., Bräutigam, A., Pick, T.R., Alter, P., Gahrtz, M., Witt, S., Fernie, A., Börnke, F., Fahnenstich, H., Bucher, M., Dresselhaus, T., Weber, A.P.M., Schreiber, F., Scholz, U., Sonnewald, U.: OPTIMAS-DW: A comprehensive transcriptomics, metabolomics, ionomics, proteomics and phenomics data resource for maize. BMC Plant Biology 12(1), e245 (2012)
3. Colmsee, C., Keller, E.R.J., Zanke, C., Senula, A., Funke, T., Oppermann, M., Weise, S., Scholz, U.: The Garlic and Shallot Core Collection image database of IPK presenting two vegetatively maintained crops in the Federal ex situ Genebank for Agricultural and Horticultural Crops at Gatersleben, Germany. Genetic Resources and Crop Evolution 59(7), 1407–1415 (2012)
4. DataCite Consortium: DataCite, http://datacite.org/ (accessed January 2014)
5. Grbavac, I., Koepler, O., Dohmeyer-Fischer, S., Fels, G., Sens, I., Brase, J.: Embedded infrastructure for primary data in chemistry. Journal of Cheminformatics 2(suppl. 1), P8 (2010)
6. Knüpffer, H., Ochsmann, J., Biermann, N.: The "Mansfeld Database" in its national and international context. Schriften zu Genetischen Ressourcen 22, 32–34 (2003)
7. Kuenne, C., Grosse, I., Matthies, I., Scholz, U., Sretenovic-Rajicic, T., Stein, N., Stephanik, A., Steuernagel, B., Weise, S.: Using Data Warehouse Technology in Crop Plant Bioinformatics. Journal of Integrative Bioinformatics 4(1), e88 (2007)

8. Künne, C., Lange, M., Funke, T., Miehe, H., Grosse, I., Scholz, U.: CR–EST: a resource for crop ESTs. Nucleic Acids Research 33(suppl.1), D619–D621 (2005)
9. Neuroth, H., Oßwald, A., Scheffel, R., Strathmann, S., Huth, K.: nestor Handbuch: Eine kleine Enzyklopädie der digitalen Langzeitarchivierung, Version 2.3 (2010), http://nestor.sub.uni-goettingen.de/handbuch/index.php (accessed January 2014)
10. Schadt, E.E., Linderman, M.D., Sorenson, J., Lee, L., Nolan, G.P.: Computational solutions to large-scale data management and analysis. Nature Reviews Genetics 11(9), 647–657 (2010)
11. Schreiber, F., Colmsee, C., Czauderna, T., Grafahrend-Belau, E., Hartmann, A., Junker, A., Junker, B.H., Klapperstück, M., Scholz, U., Weise, S.: MetaCrop 2.0: managing and exploring information about crop plant metabolism. Nucleic Acids Research 40(D1), D1173–D1177 (2012)
12. Swedlow, J.R., Zanetti, G., Best, C.: Channeling the data deluge. Nat. Methods 8(6), 463–465 (2011)
13. Thaller, M.: Das Digitale Archiv NRW in der Praxis. Verlag Dr. Kovac (2013)

A Semantic Web Faceted Search System for Facilitating Building of Biodiversity and Ecosystems Services

Marie-Angélique Laporte[1], Isabelle Mougenot[2], Eric Garnier[3], Ulrike Stahl[1,4], Lutz Maicher[1,5], and Jens Kattge[1,4]

[1] German Centre for Integrative Biodiversity Research (iDiv) Halle-Jena-Leipzig,
Deutscher Platz 5e, 04103 Leipzig, Germany
[2] UMR 228 ESPACE-DEV, Maison de la Télédétection 34093 Montpellier, France
[3] Centre d'Ecologie Fonctionnelle et Evolutive (UMR 5175), 1919 Route de Mende,
34293 Montpellier Cedex 5, France
[4] Functional Biogeography Research Group,
Max Planck Institute for Biogeochemistry, 07701 Jena, Germany
[5] Fraunhofer-Zentrum für Mittel- und Osteuropa (MOEZ), 04109 Leipzig, Germany
`marieangelique.laporte@gmail.com`, `isabelle.mougenot@ird.fr`,
`eric.garnier@cefe.cnrs.fr`, `lutz.maicher@moez.fraunhofer.de`,
`ustahl,jkattge@bgc-jena.mpg.de`

Abstract. To address biodiversity issues in ecology and to assess the consequences of ecosystem changes, large quantities of long-term observational data from multiple datasets need to be integrated and characterized in a unified way. Linked open data initiatives in ecology aim at promoting and sharing such observational data at the web-scale. Here we present a web infrastructure, named Thesauform, that fully exploits the key principles of the semantic web and associated key data standards in order to guide the scientific community of experts to collectively construct, manage, visualize and query a SKOS thesaurus. The study of a thesaurus dedicated to plant functional traits demonstrates the potential of this approach. A point of great interest is to provide each expert with the opportunity to generate new knowledge and to draw novel plausible conclusions from linked data sources. Consequently, it is required to consider both the scientific topic and the objects of interest for a community of expertise. The goal is to enable users to deal with a small number of familiar and conceptual dimensions, or in other terms, facets. In this regard, a faceted search system, based on SKOS collections and enabling thesaurus browsing according to each end-users requirements is expected to greatly enhance data discovery in the context of biodiversity studies.

Keywords: Tool, Faceted Search, Thesaurus, Semantic annotation, Functional diversity, Web of Data, Plant Trait, Controlled vocabulary, Interoperability, SKOS.

1   Introduction

Resolution of key biodiversity issues goes through continued exchanges and cooperation between related domains, such as ecology, taxonomy, genomic,

H. Galhardas and E. Rahm (Eds.): DILS 2014, LNBI 8574, pp. 50–57, 2014.
© Springer International Publishing Switzerland 2014

climatology, soil sciences, etc [1]. To address biodiversity issues, it is now widely accepted that a functional approach has strong potential. Over the last decades, trait-based research has generated huge volumes of data, within multiple contexts of observations and experiments [1]. These data sets can be obtained via very different study contexts and are often described in highly specialized terms. Numerous traits can be measured, for instance, on plants [2]. But data generated by functional ecology are only minimally reused or shared within the community, or over communities, mainly due to data heterogeneity [1]. Given these limitations, open web standards and the generation of open web standards for functional ecology would advance the integration of heterogeneous content, with the primary objective of the emergence of new knowledge.

Technologies developed under the Semantic Web initiative are particularly suitable for the sharing and the dissemination of information within a community of experts. SKOS (Simple Knowledge Organization System) [3] provides a common format to manage thesaurus adequately. The final purpose of a thesaurus is to facilitate the integration and the navigation of the information available in multiple data sources. Each SKOS thesaurus can be considered as a publicly available relevant resource on the web and can be enriched via meaningful navigation between thesauri. Linked Data initiatives put a strong emphasis on representing KOS (Knowledge Organization System) for both data discovery and data access [4]. The LOD initiative (Linked Open Data) are more and more adopted by a large panel of data providers and make publically available each day data from a wide range of disciplines including the Life Science field [5]. As a result, the LOD contains more than hundred datasets [6], which can be freely used in dozens of different contexts. The potential of each data is then fully exploited. In this regard we want to emphasize the critical importance of properly connecting observational data with each other. Defining new vocabularies based on the Semantic Web standards, as SKOS, makes them fully interoperable and allows to directly benefit from data already published in this form on the Web of Data.

In this paper, we present a complete system dedicated to the ecological community allowing it to create, manage, visualize and query a SKOS thesaurus. In the context of biodiversity studies, the TOP (Trait of Plants) thesaurus [7] is used to semantically annotate scientific data managed through heterogeneous data sources, such as the TRY database [8] or the Plant Ontology (PO) [9]. The TOP thesaurus is then exploited through a faceted search engine that reflects community interests and preferences, to facilitate the appropriation of the TOP thesaurus by various end-users. The facets act also as access points on the interrelated data sources in guiding their navigation. In this paper, we foccussed on how end-user points of view can be developed and implemented.

This article is organized as follow:

- Section 2 quickly introduces the approach driven with the Thesauform tool to build the TOP thesaurus as a collaborative product, and presents how the faceted search enhances the information retrieval in ecology and beyond this.

- Section 3 explains how the thesaurus is used for integration purposes. The TOP thesaurus aggregates data from disseminated datasources with the purpose of both enriching and facilitating data interpretation.

- Finally, section 4 summarizes and discusses the strengths of our approach and refers to future works.

2   Faceted Search to Improve Information Retrieval in Ecology

In order to build a collective thesaurus, our previous work focused on the development of a tool, named Thesauform, dedicated to assist domain experts in this task. The Thesauform tool fully relies on semantic web standards, while providing a flexible and user-friendly environment for domain experts. Twenty different experts from the functional plant trait community has used the Thesauform tool to describe the different functional plant traits in use in the domain. For instance, the widely used trait "Specific Leaf Area", also known under the abbreviation SLA, is defined as "the one sided area of a fresh leaf divided by its oven-dry mass" in Cornelissen et al. 2003, and its measurement unit is expressed in meter squared by kilogram of dry mass (m2kg-1[DM]). In the thesaurus, this trait is linked to different other traits. Indeed, it falls under the broader concept of Morphology and it is related to the Leaf Blade Thickness and the Leaf Mass per Area concepts. The TOP thesaurus can be used as a bibliographic resource about plant traits information, since it is available as a web resource[1]. The TOP thesaurus fulfills its initial role to provide a standard vocabulary available to the functional ecology community, and extends beyond the basic needs to ease information retrieval. During the thesaurus building steps, many users complained about the hierarchical structure of the thesaurus, arguing that the concepts should be ordered in a different way, and even that the thesaurus should present different hierarchies. Indeed, in some cases, users were not able to find quickly and easily the concepts on which they wanted to work on. In this context, a system considering end-user points of view has been developed and offers a faceted search engine.

Classic semantic search engines based on controlled terms have been widely used to query data in the life science fields. For instance, Bioportal[2] is a web portal providing the interrogation of multiple ontologies or controlled vocabularies based on controlled terms. Although this kind of search mechanism offers a first control over the terms used for the search, it suffers from limitations since it can be difficult for an inexperienced end-user to find the relevant controlled terms to use [10]. Indeed, with classic semantic search engines, controlled terms are most of the time displayed through an auto-completed search field. This would suggest that the user has a prior knowledge of the content of the data model to query. Furthermore, information cannot always fit into a well-defined hierarchy

---

[1] http://trait_ontology.cefe.cnrs.fr:8080/Thesauform/vizIndex.jsp (developed as a proof of concepts).

[2] http://bioportal.bioontology.org/

that users know how to browse [11]. To overcome these limitations, a well known searching and filtering technique coming from the field of Information Retrieval, the faceted search, is widely used over the web.

The faceted search is an interesting solution as it facilitates the thesaurus appropriation by the end-users by helping users to define their search needs [12,10]. In this context, facets will lead to translate the vague query that a user can have, to a precise query in the system. The MUMIA [3] web site gives a simple definition of faceted search (also called faceted navigation or faceted browsing). Faceted search is "a technique for accessing a collection of information, allowing users to explore by filtering available information. A faceted classification system allows the assignment of multiple classifications to an object, enabling the classifications to be ordered in multiple ways, rather than in a single, pre-determined, taxonomic order". In other terms, each facet typically corresponds to the common features shared by a set of objects. These features are used to filter the results. Finally, in such search engines, the user is guided (no dead-end query) as the results are filtered using relevant parameters or categories, each category reflecting both the need of users in the thesaurus navigation environment and structuring the information so others can find it.

In the TOP thesaurus, five facets have been defined according to users feedbacks with the first purpose of facilitating information retrieval. In thesaurus or in any other controlled vocabulary or ontology, concepts can be assembled into semantically meaningful groups that will correspond to facets. Since facets are closely linked to both thesaurus visualization and thesaurus restitution, and not to thesaurus structure or to the information it carries, existing good practices recommend to define facets as skos:collection [13], gathering concepts with common features. The use of skos:collection allows thus to combine concepts regarding a specific subject independently of the hierarchical classification of concepts in the concept scheme. An example of facets is described in Figure 1. The functional plant trait concept Specific Leaf Area (SLA) is classified under the concept of Morphology in the thesaurus, since this trait refers to the morphology of a plant. In Figure 1, SLA is grouped with the concepts Leaf Phenology and Leaf Lifespan, because these three concepts share the common feature of being measured on the same plant part, the leaf. But Specific Leaf Area may also be classified with the Xylem Area concept, because these two measurements refer to a size measurement, the area. The categories plant organ and measurement type can then be considered as two access points to query the thesaurus by organizing the thesaurus in two different ways. Each user can then choose which access point to use to query the thesaurus according to his own preferences. The organization of the thesaurus concepts into different views corresponding to different hierarchies makes perfect sense during the user query, the reorganization of the thesaurus information facilitating the navigation in the thesaurus.

We conclude that a faceted search system is suitable to assist users in their information retrieval. Developing such a system based on facets allows to guide the consultation of datasets in an intuitive way for the user. As the TOP thesarus

---

[3] http://www.mumia-network.eu/index.php/working-groups/wg4

```
:OrganFacet   a skos:Collection;        :SizeFacet   a skos:Collection;
    skos:member :Leaf;                      skos:member :Area;
    skos:member :Root;                      skos:member :Length;
    ...                                     skos:member :Density;
    skos:member :Seed;                      skos:member :Mass;
    skos:member :Flower .                   skos:member :Volume.
:Leaf   a skos:Collection;              :Area   a skos:Collection;
    skos:member :LeafArea;                  skos:member :LeafArea;
    skos:member :Specific Leaf              skos:member :Specific Leaf
    Area;                                   Area;
    ...                                     ...
    skos:member :LeafLifespan .             skos:member :XylemArea .
```

Fig. 1. Example of facets represented in Turtle format (RDF serialization format). Two facets are presented. The Organ facet allows to query the thesaurus using a plant organ. The Size facet is used to query the thesaurus according to the type of measure. The members of the facet values (i.e. :Leaf) come directly from the concept scheme hierarchy. The selection of Leaf from the facet Organ selects only traits measured on Leaf (belonging to the skos:Collection Leaf). Then, by selecting Area from the Size facet, the results are refreshed to contain only traits measured on Leaf and measuring an Area: LeafLifespan and XylemArea are then deleted from the results list.

is used as an access point to disseminate information, data sources semantically annotated with its concepts will be able to benefit from faceted search engines as well.

3   Facets for Facilitating the Access to Disseminated Data

The TOP thesaurus serves as a stable reference resource by organizing traits and their information. It extends beyond the users needs by linking information about traits to different available data sources with the great advantage of both enriching and facilitating the data interpretation, which requires information from different domains. Consequently, TOP thesaurus concepts have been linked to two different data sources, the TRY database, the biggest functional plant traits database, and the Plant Ontology (PO), the reference controlled vocabulary describing plant entities. A real advantage of SKOS is to provide properties dedicated to the establishment of cross-references between thesauri. The mappings between the TOP thesaurus and TRY and PO relies on SKOS properties dedicated on this purpose: the exactMatch and relatedMatch properties. The mappings to both TRY and PO have been managed automatically, based on term similarity. However, for TRY, the proposed mappings have been then manually curated by an expert in order to be validated. For TRY, only the exact matches has been saved in the mapping file. For PO, as plant entities are not traits, the matches have been recorded as related matches in the mapping file using the relatedMatch property.

The benefit of linking TOP thesaurus concepts to TRY is twofold. First, the mapping TOP/TRY allows to unify the access to TRY data, managing the terms' heterogeneity used to describe TRY data. The TRY database can then take full advantage of the different semantic search engines set up to query the TOP thesaurus information. Secondly, such a mapping will enrich and complete the information of the thesaurus itself by adding meta-information coming directly from the TRY database. For instance, on the given trait information webpage, in addition of the trait information themselves (preferred term, definition, synonyms,..), the TRY observation number, the geo-referenced observation number, the number of different species on which the given trait has been measured are also displayed. This information can be useful for the user that will be then able to get indications on the community interest for the given trait and the number of available data on that specific trait.

The mappings established between the TOP concepts and the PO concepts allow assigning a reference for the plant entities cited in most of TOP trait definitions. For instance, the definition of the Specific Leaf Area does not need then to explicit what is actually a leaf. This part of the definition is provided by the PO mapping as PO clearly defined what is a leaf. Moreover, such a mapping approach will be highly beneficial to link data used in ecology or agronomy to data used in genomics following a Linked Data approach. As the TOP thesaurus is mainly used by the ecology community and PO is mainly used in the genomic field, the mapping established between PO and TOP provides the opportunity to serve as a first unifying component between the ecological and the genomic world, both of high interest in biodiversity studies.

The resulting semantic web-infrastructure is displayed in Fig. 2. The TOP thesaurus addresses the need of organizing the available information in a unifying way in a context of biodiversity studies. Indeed, the thesaurus aggregates data from different data sources in order to build new biodiversity models where the faceted system tied to the thesaurus plays a great role. Facets can be now used to access information from these relevant and disseminated data through the thesaurus, with a reorganization of the information. In fact, TRY and PO are queried through the facets and no more through the original way the information was structured. The ecological community has therefore a full-integrated access to disseminated sources in a way that reflects their interests, thus facilitating both their discovery and their reuse.

The trait information coming from the TOP thesaurus will be mainly accessed by experts from the ecology domain. Considering this, as a proof of concepts, we based our work on a user-friendly and easy to use interface, to assist experts in their access and retrieval of pertinent information. We implemented a thin-client/application server architecture using the J2EE platform, with the system application server being deployed on Apache Tomcat. We used the Jena API to manage the aspects related to the manipulation of the SKOS thesaurus. A unique aspect of our work is the implementation of a faceted search engine based on skos collections. This enhances the semantic search of trait by providing the opportunity to the user to choose his own filters.

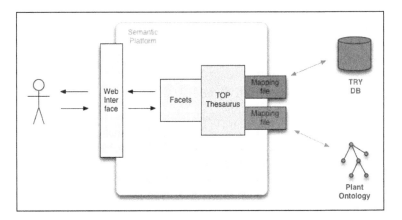

Fig. 2. Unifying system of plant trait modelling, based on Semantic Web technologies. The TOP thesaurus aggregates data from the TRY database and the Plant Ontology with the purpose of both enriching and facilitating data interpretation. The faceted search system is used to query the linked data and filter the results according to users preferences.

4   Conclusion and Perspectives

Recent studies highlight the crucial need to dispose thesaurus in the field of biodiversity and more precisely in the field of plant diversity [14,15]. Plant trait research is complex and requires information from different domains to fully exploit plant trait data. Consequently, we propose a complete system designed to the needs of the plant trait community. Such a system provides a tool to build a SKOS thesaurus and assists any community of experts to manage their datasets, and to interconnect them with data and data standards from related communities. In this regard we have emphasized the critical importance of properly connecting observational data with each other. The construction of a SKOS vocabulary facilitates the definition of clear semantic bridges between different data sources. The participation of experts, not only for the construction of thesauri, but also to validate the work related to semantic annotations, strengthens the proposed approach.

We argue that the end-user preferences have to be of prime importance in data access and retrieval. In this context, a faceted search engine demonstrates its full capabilities. First, facets ensure flexibility by playing an assistance role to users by reorganizing the thesaurus terms into meaningful groups. The faceted system supports users to specify their queries and then to drill down to results. Second, data sources semantically annotated with concepts coming from the TOP thesaurus can benefit from faceted search engine traits as well. As a consequence, facets are be used to discover and access disseminated information from heterogeneous data sources. A next step will be to propose mappings to more external resources, numerous relevant ontologies can be found on the NCBO BioPortal website. The approach championed in this paper has been to base our work on the continuity of the Open Linked Data initiative, based on Semantic Web techniques. Future work will be focused on how these facets could be automatically built from both existing literature and ontologies.

References

1. Michener, W.K., Jones, M.B.: Ecoinformatics: supporting ecology as a data-intensive science.. Trends in Ecology & Evolution 27(2), 85–93 (2012)
2. Kattge, J., Ogle, K., Bonisch, G., Diaz, S., Lavorel, S., Madin, J., Nadrowski, K., Nollert, S., Sartor, K., Wirth, C.: A generic structure for plant trait databases. Methods in Ecology & Evolution (2010)
3. Isaac, A., Summers, E.: SKOS Simple Knowledge Organization System Primer. W3C Technical Report (2008)
4. Panzer, M., Zeng, M.L.: Modeling classification systems in skos: some challenges and best-practice recommendations. In: International Conference on Dublin Core and Metadata Applications, p. 3 (2009)
5. Belleau, F., Nolin, M.A., Tourigny, N., Rigault, P., Morissette, J.: Bio2rdf: Towards a mashup to build bioinformatics knowledge systems. Journal of Biomedical Informatics 41(5), 706–716 (2008); Semantic Mashup of Biomedical Data
6. Heath, T., Bizer, C.: Linked data: Evolving the web into a global data space. Synthesis Lectures on the Semantic Web: Theory and Technology 1(1), 1–136 (2011)
7. Laporte, M.A., Garnier, E., et al.: Thesauform–traits: A web based collaborative tool to develop a thesaurus for plant functional diversity research. Ecological Informatics 11, 34–44 (2012)
8. Kattge, J., Díaz, S., Lavorel, S., Prentice, I., Leadley, P., et al.: TRY - a global database of plant traits. Global Change Biology 17 (2011)
9. Walls, R., Cooper, L., Elser, J., Stevenson, D.: The Plant Ontology: A Common Reference Ontology for Plants (2010), http://wiki.plantontology.org
10. Heim, P., Ertl, T., Ziegler, J.: Facet graphs: Complex semantic querying made easy. In: Aroyo, L., Antoniou, G., Hyvönen, E., ten Teije, A., Stuckenschmidt, H., Cabral, L., Tudorache, T. (eds.) ESWC 2010, Part I. LNCS, vol. 6088, pp. 288–302. Springer, Heidelberg (2010)
11. Uddin, M.N., Janecek, P.: Faceted classification in web information architecture: A framework for using semantic web tools. The Electronic Library 25(2), 219–233 (2007)
12. Hearst, M., Elliott, A., English, J., Sinha, R., Swearingen, K., Ping Yee, K.: Finding the flow in web site search. Commun. ACM (2002)
13. Brugman, H., Malaisé, V., Gazendam, L.: A web based general thesaurus browser to support indexing of television and radio programs. In: Proceedings of the 5th International Conference on Language Resources and Evaluation (LREC 2006), pp. 1488–1491 (2006)
14. Reichman, O.J., Jones, M.B., Schildhauer, M.P.: Challenges and Opportunities of Open Data in Ecology. Science 331(6018), 703–705 (2011)
15. Catapano, T., Hobern, D., Lapp, H., Morris, R.A., Morrison, N., Noy, N., Schildhauer, M., Thau, D.: Recommendations for the Use of Knowledge Organisation Systems by GBIF. Global Biodiversity (2011)

Handling Multiple Foci in Graph Databases

Jaudete Daltio[1,2] and Claudia Bauzer Medeiros[1]

[1] Institute of Computing - UNICAMP, Campinas, SP, Brazil
[2] Brazilian Agricultural Research Corporation's - EMBRAPA, Brazil
{jaudete,cmbm}@ic.unicamp.com

Abstract. Scientific research has become data-intensive and data-dependent, with distributed, multidisciplinary, teams creating and sharing their findings. Graph databases are being increasingly considered as a computational means to loosely integrate such data, in particular when relationships among data and the data itself are at the same importance level. However, a problem to be faced in this context is that of multiple *foci* – where a *focus*, here, is a perspective on the data, for a particular research team and context. This paper describes a conceptual framework for the construction of arbitrary foci on graph databases, to help solve this problem. The framework, under construction, is illustrated using examples based on needs of teams involved in biodiversity research.

Keywords: eScience, Graph Database, Focus, Views.

1 Introduction and Motivation

eScience, sometimes used as a synonym for data-intensive science [9], is characterized by joint research in computer science and other fields to support the whole research cycle – from data collection, mining, and visualization to data sharing. Biodiversity research – our target domain – is a good example of eScience. It is a multidisciplinary field that requires associating data about living beings and their habitats, constructing models to describe species' interactions and correlating different information sources. Such data includes information on environmental and ecological factors, as well as on species, and includes images, text, video and sound recordings [5], in multiple spatial and temporal scales.

Sharing and reuse of data are hampered by the heterogeneity of data and user requirements inherent to such domains. Each community applies different data extraction and processing methodologies and has distinct research perspectives and vocabularies. Several researchers have adopted graph representations (and graph database systems) as a computational means to deal with such integration challenges [11], especially in situations where relations among data and the data itself are at the same importance level [1].

However, graph database systems present limitations when it comes to creating and processing multiple perspectives of the underlying data. This paper presents our approach to these issues, which consists of a conceptual framework that allows experts to specify and construct arbitrary perspectives on top of

H. Galhardas and E. Rahm (Eds.): DILS 2014, LNBI 8574, pp. 58–65, 2014.

graph databases. This framework, under construction, takes advantage of some of our previous implementation work, in particular concerning ontology management [6]. Informally, the idea is to support a notion similar to that of database views, constructed on top of graph databases. However, our constructs go beyond standard database views.

Here, we follow the terminology we introduced in [13], and use the term *focus* for such views. Intuitively, a *focus* is a perspective of study of a given problem, where data can be restricted to one specific scale/representation, or put together objects from distinct scales. Moreover, given the same set of data, distinct foci will arise when the data is analyzed under different models, processed using focus-specific algorithms, or even visualized with particular means.

This paper has two main contributions. The first is to explore the notion of views on graph database systems, which is not yet supported in such systems. This requires extending the traditional specification of views, while at the same time maintaining the same principles. The second contribution is to show, via the running example, how to model and create multiple foci, for biodiversity research, thereby allowing experts to manage and analyze the same underlying datasets under arbitrary perspectives.

2   Theoretical Foundations and Related Work

2.1   Graph Databases

Graph databases allow to represent information about the connectivity of unstructured data – a recurrent scenario in scientific research. The interpretation of scientific data usually requires the understanding about linked data, interactions with other data and topological properties about data organization.

The formal foundation of all graph data structures is based on the mathematical definition of graphs and, on top of this basic layer, several graph data structures were proposed [1,12], including features such as directed or undirected edges, labeled or unlabeled edges and hypernodes. One of the most popular structures supported by many graph database systems is the *property graph*. It tries to arrange all the features that these graph types express in a single and flexible structure through key-value pairs to describe vertex and edge characteristics, such as type, label or direction.

To manipulate these data, graph query languages can be used to [14]: (i) find vertices that satisfy a pattern; (ii) find pairs (x, y) of vertices such that there is a path from x to y whose sequence of edge labels matches some pattern; (iii) express relations among paths; (iv) compute aggregate functions based on graph properties; and (v) create new elements. Each query language has its own syntax and considers its own data structure to represent a graph.

2.2   Views

In the context of relational databases, a *view* can be regarded as a temporary relation against which database requests may be issued [7]. Views are widely used to restrict, protect or reorganize relational data. Views are built by a combination of operations applied on the underlying relations, creating alternative or composite representations of existing database objects. The sequence of operations that creates a particular view is called *view generating function*.

The concept of view is used in many data management contexts. A *view of an ontology* is a subset of the original ontology, built by the extraction of some relevant parts thereof. Tools and languages for ontologies usually take advantage of their graph structure; vertices represent classes and instances and edges represent properties, relations and class hierarchies. There are different approaches to create ontology views [10]. Some are based on query languages and others are based on guidelines to navigate through ontology concepts, using the notion of *central concept* – a class around which the view is built and that defines which elements must be part of a view. Different from databases in which a query always results in an instance set, a query on an ontology can result in a partial schema (classes, relations), an instance set or a combination of both [6].

2.3   Multifocus Research

The notion of *focus* (a perspective of study of a given problem) appears naturally in eScience. The idea behind a focus is similar to the idea of an application – each application has its own perception of the world, goal, complexity and specific requirements. For the same underlying datasets, each focus represents a perception of the data, how it can be analyzed, visualized and interpreted.

A focus allows to restrict data, manage spatial and temporal scales thereof (multiple representations) and create distinct scenarios, including the vocabulary, constraints, process and rules that should be applied to the dataset [13,15]. The same data item can be interpreted in distinct ways – a species observation, for example, could represent an organism to be analyzed in a small level of detail or, in a macro perspective, a feature of a biome.

One important problem in focus-related research is how to improve data semantics, increasing its understanding and removing ambiguity. The use of ontologies has been pointed out as a means to deal with some of these issues and used to drive data management. This notion, known as *"ontology-driven information systems"* [8], uses ontologies as a central role with impact on the main components of the system and providing multiple perspectives of the data.

3   A Framework to Generate Foci

The goal of our research is to specify and implement a framework to build and explore arbitrary foci. To achieve this purpose, we extend the traditional definition of views to represent a focus, providing a reorganization of the original data or part thereof. The framework uses graph databases as the basis of data management, taking advantage of their ability to deal with highly connected datasets, a common scenario in eScience. Since graph databases do not implement the view concept, the framework introduces extensions to existing systems.

Figure 1 gives a general overview of the framework. The interface receives a focus specification as input and provides the focus as output. Both focus and underlying databases are represented as graphs (a focus may be built combining one or more graphs). The focus specification is a text file whose content and format are still under definition, using existing graph query languages (e.g. Cypher, SPARQL [12]) and the parameters of graph algorithms. Following the figure, step (1) decomposes the focus specification to define the focus generation strategies, operators and parameters. Next, the focus is created using either a query view mechanism (2); a central concept view mechanism (3); or a combination of both.

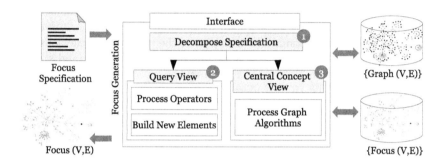

Fig. 1. Overview of the Focus Generation Process

The query view approach (2) adopts concepts from relational databases. Here we have two tasks: processing the operators that compose the query and creating new elements that do not belong to the original graph. Part of the focus specification is used to create the *"view generator function"*, the sequence of operators to be applied to the database. The traditional operators are adapted by the framework: (i) selection: to filter parts of the graph applying predicates; (ii) projection: to restrict parts of the original graph; (iii) join: to combine two or more graph databases via join conditions; (iv) aggregate functions: to provide graph summarizations, extracting vertex and edge properties.

The central concept view approach (3) is inspired by approaches to construct views on ontologies. Here, just one task is executed: processing of graph algorithms, starting from a central concept, namely a vertex defined in the focus specification. This graph algorithm can provide, for instance, the neighborhood, the shortest path to another vertex, the maximum clique, and so on [3]. The combination of these approaches allows expressiveness higher than graph query languages alone, usually untyped [4], based on triple patterns [12] and without native graph algorithms. Besides that, graph languages have limitations to create temporary elements without altering the original database and the result of a query is not necessarily a graph.

Graph databases and the foci created on the top of them are stored in a persistence layer, so that a focus can be reused. Moreover, since a focus is represented as a sub-graph, it can be used to construct other foci. We also keep the specification that originates a focus for provenance information – e.g., to describe the perspective materialized in the focus and to allow to update a focus when the graph databases used to generate it are updated.

4   Running Example

Our running example concerns biodiversity studies of animal species, concentrating on observation metadata. In particular, we deal with observations of animal vocalizations, motivated by the challenges faced by the Fonoteca Neotropical Jacques Vielliard (FNJV) at the University of Campinas (UNICAMP) [1]. FNJV has a large collection of animal sound recordings (about 30 thousand observations), whose metadata is stored in a relational database [5]. Observation metadata include information about the species, the place where the sound was recorded, the recording devices, date and time of the observation, and so on.

Although the metadata is, currently, structured as a relational database, it can be directly converted to a property graph database [12], applying straight formal approaches, e.g. [2,11]. Each row of each table can be modeled as a vertex, using the column names as attributes, and each foreign key can be modeled as an edge. Altogether, an observation has 54 metadata attributes, which can be combined in different ways to determine the edges of the graph database. Figure 2 shows one possible graph database denoted by G_{obs}. In the figure, vertices 1 through 6 represent the taxonomic hierarchy of the observed species, and vertices 8 through 11 characterize an observation, represented by vertex 7.

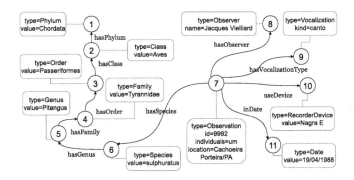

Fig. 2. Partial Metadata Graph Database of FNJV Observations - G_{obs}

G_{obs} can be integrated with many additional information sources, such as biological and environmental variables to describe the context in which vocalizations were recorded. Distinct pieces of information can be used to produce specific analyses and to build foci. A focus may concern, for example, a geographical scale or a group of species of interest. The following examples describe some use scenarios of foci for this graph database.

[1] http://proj.lis.ic.unicamp.br/fnjv

4.1   Example Focus 1: Location and Biomes

An example of focus which changes the perspective of analysis is defined as: *"Set of all locations in which observations were made, summarizing the number of distinct species observed at each location, and connecting the locations that belong to the same biome"*. This kind of focus can be helpful to analyze the biological and environmental characteristics of locations that were targets of study. To process this focus, it is necessary to aggregate the observation data to generate new information (here, the number of distinct species) and to link the original data with biome information (graph external to our database).

Let us first consider just the first part of the focus: *"Set of all locations in which observations were made, summarizing the number of distinct species observed at each location"*. This kind of focus can also be processed by the query view approach (2) of the framework, combining: (i) "build new element" operator, to create the set of vertices with type **Location** from the attribute *location* of vertices of type **Observation** in G_{bio}; (ii) "aggregate function" operator, to count the number of distinct species observed in each **Location** and store the value in *numberOfSpecies* attribute; (iii) "projection" operator, to filter the vertex and edge types that should be part of the focus (in this case, **Location**).

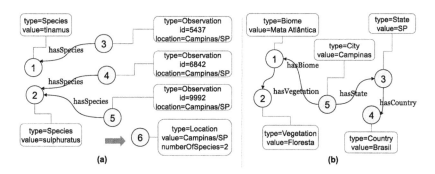

Fig. 3. Focus: (a) location and number of distinct species and (b) Partial Biome Graph Database - G_{bio}

Figure 3 (a) presents a portion of G_{obs} and explains these steps, with the creation of vertex 6 **Campinas SP** of type **Location** and *numberOfSpecies* (here, set to value 2). To connect the locations of the same biome, it is necessary to add biome information not available in G_{obs}. Figure 3 (b) shows a partial biome graph database (here shortened to G_{bio}), which is used to integrate this information, using the join operator. In this case, the focus specification combines: (i) "join" operator, to link each vertex with type **Location** in G_{obs} with the corresponding vertex of type **Biome** in G_{bio}, creating an edge (**hasBiome**) between **Location** and **Biome**; (ii) "build new element" operator, to create the set of edges with type **sameBiome** beetween the **Locations** connected to the same **Biome**; (iii) "projection" operator, to filter the vertex and edge types that

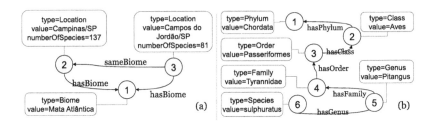

Fig. 4. (a) Query View Focus: Observation Locations and Biomes (b) Central Concept Focus: species closest to **Tinamus tao**

should be part of the focus (vertices of types **Location** and **Biome**). A partial view of the result focus is shown in Figure 4 (a).

4.2   Example Focus 2: Species "Closely Related" to Tinamus tao

Another possible scenario builds the focus from a central concept. Here, an example would be: *"Which are the species closest in the taxonomy to the species **Tinamus tao**"*. This kind of focus can be helpful to analyze the diversity of the species observed according to the "closeness" to other species within a taxonomic level (e.g. genus, family or order). This focus can be processed by the central concept view approach (3) of the framework, starting from species *Tinamus tao* in G_{obs}. The graph for this focus is built considering only edges related with taxonomic classification levels. The notion of closeness here is defined considering the distance between the vertices in G_{obs}: closest mean shortest paths.

The generating function combines: (i) "projection" operator, to filter from G_{obs} the set of vertex and edge types that should be part of the focus (in this case, vertex types related to taxonomic level); (ii) "central concept", in this case, the vertex of type **Species** that represents the species *Tinamus tao*; (iii) the graph algorithm to be applied, in this case, shortest path. The focus result contains all species vertices in the graph for which the paths to species *Tinamus tao* are minimal. A partial result focus is shown in Figure 4 (b).

This focus can be further restricted to *"Species closest in taxonomy to **Tinamus tao**, observed in the same locations"*. This can be helpful to understand the similarity among environments where "closely related" species are observed. In this case, specification of focus 2 should be extended, including a "selection" operator to filter only species observed in the same locations. This focus demands a combination of all functionalities available in the focus generation module.

5   Conclusions and Ongoing Work

This paper presented the specification of a framework to to build and explore arbitrary foci in scientific databases, using graph databases as the basis of data management. The approach extends the traditional definition of views in relational databases to represent a focus, combining graph query languages with graph algorithms to build customized foci. The internals of the framework were explained via examples in biodiversity data management, pointing out some of challenges to be faced. The implementation of the framework will take advantage of previous work of ours in ontology management [6].

The first challenge involves extending the concept of view of relational databases to graph databases. Another challenge is related to the specification of a focus. At the moment, we assume that a focus is specified by indicating a suite of operations to be applied to the underling graph databases. This, however, will need to be improved once we formalize focus construction operators.

Acknowledgements. Work partially financed by FAPESP/Cepid in Computational Engineering and Sciences, MSR FAPESP Virtual Institute (NavScales), CNPq (MuZOO), FAPESP-PRONEX (eScience), and grants from CNPq.

References

1. Angles, R., Gutierrez, C.: Survey of graph database models. ACM Comput. Surv. 40(1), 1:1–1:39 (2008)
2. Bizer, C.: D2rq - treating non-rdf databases as virtual rdf graphs. In: Proceedings of the 3rd International Semantic Web Conference (2004)
3. Brandes, U., Erlebach, T.: Network Analysis: Methodological Foundations. LNCS. Springer-Verlag New York, Inc., Secaucus (2005)
4. Colazzo, D., Sartiani, C.: Typing query languages for data graphs. In: I. W. on Graph Data Management: Techniques and Applications (2014)
5. Cugler, D.C., Medeiros, C.B., Toledo, L.F.: An architecture for retrieval of animal sound recordings based on context variables. In: Concurrency and Computation: Practice and Experience, pp. 1–17 (2011)
6. Daltio, J., Medeiros, C.B.: Aondê: An ontology web service for interoperability across biodiversity applications. Information Systems 33(7-8), 724–753 (2008)
7. Furtado, A., Sevcik, K., Santos, C.: Permitting updates through views of databases. Informations Systems 4, 269–283 (1979)
8. Guarino, N.: Formal ontology and information systems. In: Proceedings of Formal Ontology in Information System, pp. 3–15. IOS Press (1998)
9. Hey, T., Tansley, S., Tolle, K. (eds.): The Fourth Paradigm: Data-Intensive Scientific Discovery. Microsoft Research, Redmond (2009)
10. Noy, N.F., Musen, M.A.: Specifying ontology views by traversal. In: McIlraith, S.A., Plexousakis, D., van Harmelen, F. (eds.) ISWC 2004. LNCS, vol. 3298, pp. 713–725. Springer, Heidelberg (2004)
11. Park, Y., Shankar, M., Park, B., Ghosh, J.: Graph databases for large-scale healthcare systems: A framework for efficient data management and data services. In: I. W. on Graph Data Management: Techniques and Applications (2014)
12. Robinson, I., Webber, J., Eifrem, E.: Graph Databases. O'Reilly Media (2013) (Incorporated)
13. Santanche, A., Medeiros, C.B., Jomier, J., Zam, M.: Challenges of the Anthropocene epoch - Supporting multi-focus research. In: Proc XIII GeoINFO (2012)
14. Wood, P.T.: Query languages for graph databases. SIGMOD Rec. 41(1), 50–60 (2012)
15. Zhou, S., Jones, C.B.: A multi-representation spatial data model. In: Hadzilacos, T., Manolopoulos, Y., Roddick, J., Theodoridis, Y. (eds.) SSTD 2003. LNCS, vol. 2750, pp. 394–411. Springer, Heidelberg (2003)

Completing the is-a Structure of Biomedical Ontologies

Zlatan Dragisic[1,2], Patrick Lambrix[1,2], and Fang Wei-Kleiner[1]

[1] Department of Computer and Information Science, Linköping University, 581 83 Linköping,
Sweden
[2] Swedish e-Science Research Centre, Sweden

Abstract. Ontologies in the biomedical domain are becoming a key element for
data integration and search. The usefulness of the applications which use ontologies is often directly influenced by the quality of ontologies, as incorrect or
incomplete ontologies might lead to wrong or incomplete results for the applications. Therefore, there is an increasing need for repairing defects in ontologies.
In this paper we focus on completing ontologies. We provide an algorithm for
completing the is-a structure in $\mathcal{EL}$ ontologies which covers many biomedical
ontologies. Further, we present an implemented system based on the algorithm as
well as an evaluation using three biomedical ontologies.

1 Introduction

With the increasing presence of biomedical data sources on the Internet more and more
research effort is put into finding possible ways for integrating and searching such often
heterogeneous sources. Semantic Web technologies such as ontologies, are becoming
a key technology in this effort. Ontologies provide a means for modelling the domain
of interest and they allow for information reuse, portability and sharing across multiple platforms. Efforts such as the Open Biological and Biomedical Ontologies (OBO)
Foundry, BioPortal and Unified Medical Language System (UMLS) aim at providing
repositories for biomedical ontologies and relations between these ontologies thus providing means for annotating and sharing biomedical data sources. Many of the ontologies in the biomedical domain can be represented using the $\mathcal{EL}$ description logic or
small extensions thereof (e.g. [1] and the TONES Ontology Repository).

Developing ontologies is not an easy task, and often the resulting ontologies (including their is-a structures) are not complete. In addition to being problematic for the
correct modelling of a domain, such incomplete ontologies also influence the quality of
semantically-enabled applications. Incomplete ontologies when used in semantically-
enabled applications can lead to valid conclusions being missed.

In ontology-based search, queries are refined and expanded by moving up and down
the hierarchy of concepts. Incomplete structure in ontologies influences the quality
of the search results. As an example, suppose we want to find articles in the MeSH
Database of PubMed using the term *Scleral Diseases* in MeSH. By default the query
will follow the hierarchy of MeSH and include more specific terms for searching, such
as *Scleritis*. If the relation between *Scleral Diseases* and *Scleritis* is missing in MeSH,
we will miss 922 articles in the search result, which is about 57% of the original result[1]. The structural information is also important information in ontology engineering

---

[1] PubMed accessed on 21-02-2014.

H. Galhardas and E. Rahm (Eds.): DILS 2014, LNBI 8574, pp. 66–80, 2014.

research. For instance, most current ontology alignment systems use structure-based strategies to find mappings between the terms in different ontologies (e.g. overview in [27]) and the modeling defects in the structure of the ontologies have an important influence on the quality of the ontology alignment results.

In this paper we tackle the problem of completing the is-a structure of ontologies. Completing the is-a structure requires adding new correct is-a relations to the ontology. We identify two cases for finding relations which need to be added to an ontology. In **case 1** missing is-a relations have been detected and the task is to find ways of making these detected is-a relations derivable in the ontology. There are many approaches to detect missing is-a relations, e.g., using linguistic or logical patterns or by using knowledge intrinsic to an ontology network (see Section 6). However, in general, these approaches do not detect *all* missing is-a relations and in several cases even only few. Therefore, we assume that we have obtained a set of missing is-a relations for a given ontology (but not necessarily all). In the case where our set of missing is-a relations contains *all* missing is-a relations, completing the ontology is easy. We just add all missing is-a relations to the ontology and a reasoner can compute all logical consequences. However, when the set of missing is-a relations does not contain all missing is-a relations - and this is the common case - there are different ways to complete the ontology. The easiest way is still to just add the missing is-a relations to the ontology. For instance, T in Figure 1 represents a small ontology inspired by Galen ontology (http://www.co-ode.org/galen/), that is relevant for our discussions. Assume that we have detected that Endocarditis $\sqsubseteq$ PathologicalPhenomenon and GranulomaProcess $\sqsubseteq$ NonNormalProcess are missing is-a relations (M in Figure 1). Obviously, adding these relations to the ontology will repair the missing is-a structure. However, there are other more interesting possibilities. For instance, adding Carditis $\sqsubseteq$ CardioVascularDisease and GranulomaProcess $\sqsubseteq$ PathologicalProcess also repairs the missing is-a structure. Further, these is-a relations are correct according to the domain and constitute new is-a relations (e.g. Carditis $\sqsubseteq$ CardioVascularDisease) that were not derivable from the ontology and not originally detected by the detection algorithm.[2] We also note that from a logical point of view, adding Carditis $\sqsubseteq$ Fracture and GranulomaProcess $\sqsubseteq$ NonNormalProcess also repairs the missing is-a structure. However, from the point of view of the domain, this solution is not correct. Therefore, as it is the case for all approaches for dealing with modeling defects, a domain expert needs to validate the logical solutions.

In **case 2** no missing is-a relations are given. In this case we investigate existing is-a relations in the ontology and try to find new ways of deriving these existing is-a relations. This might pinpoint to the necessity of adding new missing is-a relations to the ontology. As an example, let us assume that our ontology contains relations $T \cup M$ in Figure 1. If we assume now that we want to investigate new ways of deriving relations in M then obviously adding Carditis $\sqsubseteq$ CardioVascularDisease and GranulomaProcess $\sqsubseteq$ PathologicalProcess would be one possibility given that both are correct according to the domain.

The basic problem underlying the two cases can be formalized in the same way (Section 2.2).

---

[2] Therefore, the approach in this paper can also be seen as a detection method that takes already found missing is-a relations as input.

C = { GranulomaProcess, CardioVascularDisease, PathologicalPhenomenon, Fracture, Endocarditis, Carditis, InflammationProcess, PathologicalProcess, NonNormalProcess}

T = { CardioVascularDisease $\sqsubseteq$ PathologicalPhenomenon, Fracture $\sqsubseteq$ PathologicalPhenomenon, $\exists$hasAssociatedProcess.PathologicalProcess $\sqsubseteq$ PathologicalPhenomenon, Endocarditis $\sqsubseteq$ Carditis, Endocarditis $\sqsubseteq$ $\exists$hasAssociatedProcess.InflammationProcess, PathologicalProcess $\sqsubseteq$ NonNormalProcess }

M = { Endocarditis $\sqsubseteq$ PathologicalPhenomenon, GranulomaProcess $\sqsubseteq$ NonNormalProcess }

The following is-a relations are correct according to the domain, i.e., Or returns $true$ for:
GranulomaProcess $\sqsubseteq$ InflammationProcess, GranulomaProcess $\sqsubseteq$ PathologicalProcess,
GranulomaProcess $\sqsubseteq$ NonNormalProcess, CardioVascularDisease $\sqsubseteq$ PathologicalPhenomenon,
Fracture $\sqsubseteq$ PathologicalPhenomenon, Endocarditis $\sqsubseteq$ PathologicalPhenomenon,
Endocarditis $\sqsubseteq$ Carditis, Endocarditis $\sqsubseteq$ CardioVascularDisease, Carditis $\sqsubseteq$ PathologicalPhenomenon,
Carditis $\sqsubseteq$ CardioVascularDisease, InflammationProcess $\sqsubseteq$ PathologicalProcess,
InflammationProcess $\sqsubseteq$ NonNormalProcess, PathologicalProcess $\sqsubseteq$ NonNormalProcess.

Let $\mathcal{P}$ = GTAP(T, C, Or, M).

Fig. 1. Small example

The contributions of this paper are the following. We present an approach for completing the is-a structure of $\mathcal{EL}$ ontologies which aims at introducing new information to the ontology (Section 3). Together with the algorithm for completing the is-a structure we present an implemented system (Section 4). Next, we provide an evaluation of the system using three ontologies from the biomedical domain and discuss lessons learned. The paper concludes with the discussion of related work and possible future work (Sections 6 and 7). We continue with some necessary preliminaries in Section 2.

2   Preliminaries

2.1   The Description Logic $\mathcal{EL}$

Concept descriptions are constructed inductively from a set N_C of atomic concepts and a set N_R of atomic roles. The concept constructors are the top concept $\top$, conjunction, and existential restriction. The syntax of the different constructors can be found in Figure 2. An interpretation $\mathcal{I}$ consists of a non-empty set $\Delta^{\mathcal{I}}$ and an interpretation function $\cdot^{\mathcal{I}}$ which assigns to each atomic concept $A \in N_C$ a subset $A^{\mathcal{I}} \subseteq \Delta^{\mathcal{I}}$, to each atomic role $r \in N_R$ a relation $r^{\mathcal{I}} \subseteq \Delta^{\mathcal{I}} \times \Delta^{\mathcal{I}}$. The interpretation function is straightforwardly extended to complex concepts. An $\mathcal{EL}$ TBox[3] is a finite set of *general concept inclusions* (GCIs), whose syntax can be found in the lower part of Figure 2. An interpretation $\mathcal{I}$ is a *model* of a TBox T if for each GCI in T, the conditions given in the third column of Figure 2 are satisfied.

The main reasoning task for description logics is subsumption in which the problem is to decide for a TBox T and concepts C and D whether $T \models C \sqsubseteq D$. Subsumption in $\mathcal{EL}$ is polynomial.

---

[3] Named CBox in [1].

Name	Syntax	Semantics
top	$\top$	$\Delta^{\mathcal{I}}$
conjunction	$C \sqcap D$	$C^{\mathcal{I}} \cap D^{\mathcal{I}}$
existential restriction	$\exists r.C$	$\{x \in \Delta^{\mathcal{I}} \mid \exists y \in \Delta^{\mathcal{I}} : (x,y) \in r^{\mathcal{I}} \wedge y \in C^{\mathcal{I}}\}$
GCI	$C \sqsubseteq D$	$C^{\mathcal{I}} \subseteq D^{\mathcal{I}}$

Fig. 2. $\mathcal{EL}$ Syntax and Semantics

2.2 Completing is-a Structure

The problem of completing the missing is-a structure in an ontology can be formalized as a generalized version of the TBox abduction problem [28].

We assume that our ontology is represented using a TBox T in $\mathcal{EL}$. Further, we have a set of missing is-a relations which are represented by a set M of atomic concept subsumptions. In *case 1* in the introduction, these missing is-a relations were detected. In *case 2* the elements in M are existing is-a relations in the ontology that are temporarily removed, and T represents the ontology that is obtained by removing the elements in M from the original ontology. (They can later be added again after completing the ontology.) To complete the is-a structure of an ontology, the ontology should be extended with a set S of atomic concept subsumptions (repair) such that the extended ontology entails the missing is-a relations. However, the added atomic concept subsumptions should be correct according to the domain. In general, the set of all atomic concept subsumptions that are correct according to the domain are not known beforehand. Indeed, if this set were given then we would only have to add this to the ontology. The common case, however, is that we do not have this set, but instead can rely on a domain expert that can decide whether an atomic concept subsumption is correct according to the domain. In our formalization the domain expert is represented by an oracle Or that when given an atomic concept subsumption, returns true or false. It is then required that for every atomic concept subsumption $s \in S$, we have that $Or(s) = true$. The following definition formalizes this.

Definition 1 (Generalized TBox Abduction). *(variant of [28])*
Let T be a TBox in $\mathcal{EL}$ and C be the set of all atomic concepts in T.
Let $M = \{A_i \sqsubseteq B_i \mid A_i, B_i \in C\}$ be a finite set of TBox assertions.
Let $Or : \{C_i \sqsubseteq D_i \mid C_i, D_i \in C\} \rightarrow \{true, false\}$.
A solution to the generalized TBox abduction problem (GTAP) (T, C, Or, M) is any finite set $S = \{E_i \sqsubseteq F_i \mid E_i, F_i \in C \wedge Or(E_i \sqsubseteq F_i) = true\}$ of TBox assertions, such that $T \cup S$ is consistent and $T \cup S \models M$.

We note that an additional condition could be enforced in the definition i.e. $\forall m \in M : Or(m) = true$. Regarding this condition, if some missing is-a relation is not correct according to the domain, it could still be possible to find a solution. However, in this case the domain expert makes mistakes in the judgement or T is not correct according to the domain. In practice, it is therefore advantageous to validate whether the missing is-a relations are correct according to the domain before repairing.

As an example, let us consider GTAP $\mathcal{P}$ as defined in Figure 1. Then a possible solution for $\mathcal{P}$ is {Carditis $\sqsubseteq$ CardioVascularDisease, InflammationProcess $\sqsubseteq$ PathologicalProcess, GranulomaProcess $\sqsubseteq$ InflammationProcess}. Another possible solution is {Carditis $\sqsubseteq$ CardioVascularDisease, GranulomaProcess $\sqsubseteq$ PathologicalProcess} as explained in Section 1.

There can be many solutions for a GTAP and, as explained in Section 1, not all solutions are equally interesting. Therefore, in [28] we proposed two preference criteria on the solutions. The first criterion is a criterion that is not used in other abduction problems, but that is particularly important for GTAP. In GTAP it is important to find solutions that add to the ontology as much information as possible that is correct according to the domain. Therefore, the first criterion prefers solutions that imply more information.

Definition 2 (More Informative). *Let S and S' be two solutions to the GTAP (T, C, Or, M). S is said to be* more informative *than S' iff $T \cup S \models S'$ and $T \cup S' \not\models S$.*

Further, we say that S is equally informative *as S' iff $T \cup S \models S'$ and $T \cup S' \models S$.*

Consider two solutions[4] to $\mathcal{P}$, S_1 = {InflammationProcess $\sqsubseteq$ PathologicalProcess, GranulomaProcess $\sqsubseteq$ InflammationProcess} and S_2 = {InflammationProcess $\sqsubseteq$ PathologicalProcess, GranulomaProcess $\sqsubseteq$ PathologicalProcess}. In this case solution S_1 is more informative than S_2.

The second criterion is a classical criterion in abduction problems. It requires that no element in a solution is redundant.

Definition 3 (Subset Minimality). *A solution S to the GTAP (T, C, Or, M) is said to be subset minimal iff there is no proper subset $S' \subsetneq S$ such that S' is a solution.*

An example of a subset minimal solution for $\mathcal{P}$ is {InflammationProcess $\sqsubseteq$ PathologicalProcess, GranulomaProcess $\sqsubseteq$ InflammationProcess}. On the other hand, solution {Carditis $\sqsubseteq$ CardioVascularDisease, InflammationProcess $\sqsubseteq$ PathologicalProcess, GranulomaProcess $\sqsubseteq$ InflammationProcess} is not subset minimal as it contains Carditis $\sqsubseteq$ CardioVascularDisease which is redundant for repairing the missing is-a relations.

Three different combinations of these criteria were identified and formalized in [28]. Solutions with higher level of informativeness and no redundancy are preferred and this is formalized by skyline optimality.

Definition 4 (Skyline Optimal). *A solution S to the GTAP (T, C, Or, M) is said to be skyline optimal iff there does not exist another solution S' such that S' is a proper subset of S and S' is equally informative as S.*

---

[4] Observe that both missing is-relations are derivable using S_1. GranulomaProcess $\sqsubseteq$ NonNormalProcess is derivable as GranulomaProcess $\sqsubseteq$ InflammationProcess (S_1), InflammationProcess $\sqsubseteq$ PathologicalProcess (S_1), and PathologicalProcess $\sqsubseteq$ NonNormalProcess (T). Endocarditis $\sqsubseteq$ PathologicalPhenomenon is derivable as Endocarditis $\sqsubseteq$ $\exists$hasAssociatedProcess.InflammationProcess (T), $\exists$hasAssociatedProcess.InflammationProcess $\sqsubseteq$ $\exists$hasAssociatedProcess.PathologicalProcess (S_1), and $\exists$hasAssociatedProcess.PathologicalProcess $\sqsubseteq$ PathologicalPhenomenon (T). Similarly for S_2.

For example, {InflammationProcess $\sqsubseteq$ PathologicalProcess, GranulomaProcess $\sqsubseteq$ InflammationProcess, Carditis $\sqsubseteq$ CardioVascularDisease} is a skyline optimal solution for $\mathcal{P}$.

3   Algorithm

In this section we present an algorithm for completing the is-a structure (solving GTAP (T, C, Or, M)) in ontologies that are represented in $\mathcal{EL}$ and where the TBox is normalized as described in [1]. A normalized TBox T contains only axioms of the forms $A_1 \sqcap \ldots \sqcap A_n \sqsubseteq B$, $A \sqsubseteq \exists r.B$, and $\exists r.A \sqsubseteq B$, where $A, A_1, \ldots, A_n$ and B are atomic concepts and r is a role. Further, based on lessons learned in [28], we require that the missing is-a relations are validated before the repairing and thus $\forall m \in M : Or(m) = true$. This, together with the fact that $\mathcal{EL}$ TBoxes are always consistent, gives us that M is a solution.

In general, we would like to find a solution for GTAP at the highest level of informativeness. However, this can only be *guaranteed* if we know *all* missing is-a relations. One way to obtain this is using a brute-force method and ask Or for every pair in $C \times C$ whether it is a correct is-a relation according to the domain or not. In practice, for large ontologies this is not feasible. Therefore, the algorithm in Algorithm 1 computes initially a skyline optimal solution for GTAP (T, C, Or, M) and iteratively tries to find other skyline optimal solutions at higher levels of informativeness. As M is a solution, the algorithm will always return a result. The result can be a subset minimal solution that is a subset of M or a solution that is more informative than M.

The basic step in the algorithm (*RepairSingleIsa*) computes a solution for a GTAP with one missing is-a relation (i.e. GTAP $(T, C, Or, \{E \sqsubseteq F\})$) in the following way. First, superconcepts of E are collected in a *Source* set and subconcepts of F are collected in a *Target* set (lines 3 and 4). *Source* contains expressions of the forms A and $\exists r.A$ while *Target* contains expressions of the forms A, $A_1 \sqcap \ldots \sqcap A_n$ and $\exists r.A$ where A, $A_1, \ldots, A_n$ are atomic concepts and r is a role. Adding an is-a relation between an element in Source and an element in Target to the ontology would make $E \sqsubseteq F$ derivable (and thus this gives us logical solutions, but not necessarily solutions that are correct according to the domain). As we are interested in solutions containing is-a relations between atomic concepts, we check for every pair (A,B) $\in$ Source $\times$ Target whether A and B are atomic concepts and $Or(A \sqsubseteq B) = true$ (i.e. correct according to the domain). If so, then this is a possible solution for GTAP $(T, C, Or, \{E \sqsubseteq F\})$. However, if the current solution already contains is-a relations that would lead to the entailment of $A \sqsubseteq B$ then we do not use $A \sqsubseteq B$ (8-9). Otherwise we use $A \sqsubseteq B$ and remove elements from the current solution that would be entailed if $A \sqsubseteq B$ is used (10-12). Further, in the case where A is of the form $\exists r.N$ and B is of the form $\exists r.O$, then making $N \sqsubseteq O$ derivable would also make $A \sqsubseteq B$ derivable (13-14). It is clear that for the result of *RepairSingleIsa*, i.e. Sol, the following holds: $T \cup Sol \models E \sqsubseteq F$ and $\forall s \in Sol : Or(s) = true$. Together with the fact that $\mathcal{EL}$ TBoxes are consistent, this leads to the fact that Sol is a solution of GTAP $(T, C, Or, \{E \sqsubseteq F\})$.

In *RepairMultipleIsa* the algorithm collects for each missing is-a relation a solution from *RepairSingleIsa* and takes the union of these. Therefore, the following holds for

```
 1  Procedure RepairSingleIsa begin
        Input: E ⊑ F, T, Or, C
        Output: Solution for GTAP (T, C, Or, {E ⊑ F})
 2      Sol := ∅;
 3      Source := find superconcepts of E;
 4      Target := find subconcepts of F;
 5      foreach A ∈ Source do
 6          foreach B ∈ Target do
 7              if A and B are atomic concepts & A ⊑ B ∈ Or then
 8                  if there exists K ⊑ L ∈ Sol such that T ⊨ A ⊑ K and T ⊨ L ⊑ B then
 9                      do nothing;
10                  else
11                      remove every K ⊑ L ∈ Sol s.t. T ⊨ K ⊑ A and T ⊨ B ⊑ L;
12                      Sol := Sol ∪ {A ⊑ B};
13              else if A is of the form ∃r.N & B is of the form ∃r.O then
14                  Sol := Sol ∪ RepairSingleIsa(N ⊑ O, T, Or, C);
15      return Sol;

16  Procedure RepairMultipleIsa begin
        Input: M, T, Or, C
        Output: Solution for GTAP (T, C, Or, M)
17      foreach E_i ⊑ F_i ∈ M do
18          SingleSol_i := RepairSingleIsa(E_i ⊑ F_i, T, Or, C);
19      Solution := ⋃_i SingleSol_i;
20      remove redundancy in Solution within same level of informativeness;
21      return Solution;

22  Procedure Repair begin
        Input: M, T, Or, C
        Output: Solution for GTAP (T, C, Or, M)
23      Missing := M;
24      Solution := RepairMultipleIsa(Missing, T, Or, C);
25      Final-Solution := Solution;
26      while Solution ≠ Missing do
27          Missing := Solution;
28          Solution := RepairMultipleIsa(Missing, T ∪ Missing, Or, C);
29          Final-Solution := Final-Solution ∪ Solution;
30          remove redundancy in Final-Solution within same level of informativeness;
31      return Final-Solution;
```

Algorithm 1. Solving GTAP

Solution in line 19: $T \cup Solution \models M$ and $\forall s \in Solution : Or(s) = true$. Together with the fact that $\mathcal{EL}$ TBoxes are consistent, this leads to the fact that Solution is a solution of GTAP (T, C, Or, M). Further, in line 20, we remove redundancy while keeping the same level of informativeness, and thus obtain a skyline optimal solution. (In the case where there are several ways to remove redundancy, one is chosen, as the extended ontologies will be equivalent in the sense that they entail the same statements.)

In *Repair* we try to improve the result from *RepairMultipleIsa* by trying to find a skyline optimal solution at a higher level of informativeness. Given that any element in the solution of *RepairMultipleIsa* that is not in M can be considered as a new missing is-a relation (which was not detected earlier), we can try to find additional more informative ways of repairing by solving a new GTAP problem for these new missing is-a relations (and continue as long as new missing is-a relations are detected). As a (skyline optimal) solution for the new GTAP is also a (skyline optimal) solution of the original GTAP, the solution found in *Repair* is a skyline optimal solution for the original GTAP.

As an example run consider the GTAP in Figure 1. For a given ontology and set of missing is-a relations, the algorithm will first find solutions for repairing individual missing is-a relations using *RepairSingleIsA*. For the missing is-a relation Endocarditis ⊑ PathologicalPhenomenon the following is-a relations provide logical solutions for repairing the missing is-a relation: Endocarditis ⊑ PathologicalPhenomenon, Endocarditis ⊑ Fracture, Endocarditis ⊑ CardioVascularDisease, Carditis ⊑ PathologicalPhenomenon, Carditis ⊑ Fracture, Carditis ⊑ CardioVascularDisease as well as InflammationProcess ⊑ PathologicalProcess. As the first one is the missing is-a relation which was already validated, only the other six is-a relations are presented to the oracle for validation. Out of these six Endocarditis ⊑ Fracture and Carditis ⊑ Fracture are not correct according to the domain and are therefore not included in solutions. Further, relations Endocarditis ⊑ CardioVascularDisease, Endocarditis ⊑ PathologicalPhenomenon, Carditis ⊑ PathologicalPhenomenon are removed given it is possible to entail them from the ontology together with the remaining relations. Therefore, after validation, *RepairSingleIsA* returns {InflammationProcess ⊑ PathologicalProcess, Carditis ⊑ CardioVascularDisease}. The same process is repeated for the second missing is-a relation GranulomaProcess ⊑ NonNormalProcess. In this case the following is-a relations provide logical solutions for repairing the missing is-a relation: GranulomaProcess ⊑ NonNormalProcess and GranulomaProcess ⊑ PathologicalProcess. GranulomaProcess ⊑ NonNormalProcess is the missing is-a relation and was already validated as correct according to the domain. GranulomaProcess ⊑ PathologicalProcess is presented to the oracle and validated as correct according to the domain. As GranulomaProcess ⊑ NonNormalProcess can be entailed from the ontology together with GranulomaProcess ⊑ PathologicalProcess, *RepairSingleIsA* returns {GranulomaProcess ⊑ PathologicalProcess}. The solutions for the single is-a relations are then combined to form a solution for the set of missing is-a relations. In our case, there are no redundant relations and therefore *RepairMultipleIsA* returns {InflammationProcess ⊑ PathologicalProcess, Carditis ⊑ CardioVascularDisease, GranulomaProcess ⊑ PathologicalProcess}. We note that this is a skyline optimal solution. In *Repair* the system tries to improve the acquired solution. This time the oracle is presented with a total of 13 relations for validation out of which only one is validated to be correct, i.e. GranulomaProcess ⊑ InflammationProcess. This is added to the solution. Given this new is-a relation, GranulomaProcess ⊑ PathologicalProces is removed from the solution as it can now be entailed from the ontology and GranulomaProcess ⊑ InflammationProcess. The new solution is {InflammationProcess ⊑ PathologicalProcess, Carditis ⊑ CardioVascularDisease, GranulomaProcess ⊑ InflammationProcess}. This is again a skyline optimal solution and it is more informative than the previous solution. As new missing is-a relations were detected, the repairing is run for the third time. However, in this run the solution is not improved and thus the algorithm outputs the final result. We note that in this example we found a skyline optimal solution that is also solution with the highest level of informativeness. In general, however, it is not possible to know whether the solution is of the highest level of informativeness without checking every possible is-a relation between atomic concepts in the ontology.

4   System

We have implemented a system for completing the missing is-a structure in $\mathcal{EL}$ ontologies based on the algorithm in Algorithm 1. The input to the system is a an ontology and a set of validated missing is-a relations. The output is a solution to GTAP (called

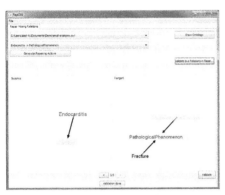
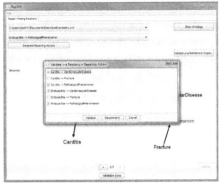

(a) Repairing using Source and Target sets.   (b) Validating is-a relations in a repairing action.

Fig. 3. System screenshots

a *repairing action*). The system was implemented in Java and uses the ELK reasoner (version 0.4.1) [21] to detect implicit entailments in the ontology. The system is semi-automatic and requires interaction with a user which is a domain expert serving as an oracle and who decides whether an is-a relation is correct according to the domain.

Once the ontology and the set of missing is-a relations are loaded, the user starts the debugging process by pressing the button `Generate Repairing Actions`. The system then removes redundant is-a relations and the non-redundant missing is-a relations are shown in a drop-down list allowing the user to switch between missing is-a relations. Additional relations acquired from lines 13 and 14 in the algorithm (Algorithm 1) are also included in the drop-down list. It is also possible to scroll between relations using the arrow buttons in the bottom part of the screen.

After selecting an is-a relation from the list, the user is presented with the Source and the Target set for that is-a relation. The user then needs to choose relations which are correct according to the domain for that is-a relation. Missing is-a relations are automatically validated to be correct according to the domain while the relations that were acquired from lines 13 and 14 in the algorithm have to be explicitly validated by the user.

In Figure 3(a) the user is presented with the Source and the Target set for the missing is-a relation Endocarditis $\sqsubseteq$ PathologicalPhenomenon (concepts in the missing is-a relation are marked in red). In this case the user has selected {Carditis $\sqsubseteq$ CardioVascularDisease} as a repairing action for the missing is-a relation (concepts marked in purple) and needs to confirm this by clicking the `Validate` button.

The user also has the option to check which relations have been validated so far and which relations can be validated, by clicking the `Validate Is-a Relations` button. In the pop-up window that appears the user can validate new relations, remove validations from already validated relations as well as ask for a recommendation by clicking the `Recommend` button (Figure 3(b)). Recommendations are acquired by querying external sources (currently, WordNet, UMLS Methathesaurus and Uberon).

The validation phase is ended by clicking on the `Validation Done` button. The system then calculates the consequences of the chosen repairing actions and presents the user with a new set of is-a relations that need to be repaired. The validation phase and consequent computations represent one iteration of the Repair procedure in Algorithm 1. If the repairing did not change between two iterations the system outputs the repairing.

At any point the user can save validated relations from the "File" menu which makes it possible to do debugging accross multiple sessions.

5   Experiments

We have run several experiments on an Intel Core i7-2620M Processor at 3.07 GHz with 4 GB RAM under Windows 7 Professional and Java 1.7 compiler. The experiments cover the two cases from the introduction. In all experiments the validation phase took the most time while the computations between iterations took less than 10 seconds.

The results are summarized in Figures 4 - 5. The 'It' columns represent the different iterations of Repair in Algorithm 1. The 'Missing' rows give the number of missing is-a relations in each iteration. Such a missing is-a relation can be repaired by adding itself ('Repaired by itself'), by adding other is-a relations that were not derivable in the ontology and thus represent new knowledge added to the ontology ('Repaired using new knowledge'). The 'New relations' row shows how many new is-a relations were added to the ontology. When such relations were found using $\exists$ (lines 13 and 14 in the algorithm), then the number of such relations is shown in parentheses. We note that for iteration $i + 1$ the number of missing is-a relations is the number of new relations from iteration i plus the number of missing is-a relations repaired by themselves from iteration i if there are no redundant relations. We also note that in the *last* iteration all missing is-a relations from that iteration are always repaired by themselves and these represent the final repairing action.

5.1   Case 1 Experiment – OAEI Anatomy

We debugged the two ontologies from the Anatomy track at the 2013 Ontology Alignment Evaluation Initiative, i.e. Mouse Anatomy ontology (AMA) containing 2744 concepts and a fragment of NCI human anatomy ontology (NCI-A) containing 3304 concepts. The input missing is-a relations for these two experiments were a set of 94 and 58 missing is-a relations, respectively, for AMA and NCI-A. These missing is-a relations were obtained by using a logic-based approach using an alignment between AMA and NCI-A [25] to generate candidate missing is-a relations which were then validated by a domain expert to obtain actual missing is-a relations. Therefore, this experiment is related to *case 1*.

Mouse Anatomy. The results for debugging AMA are given in Figure 4(a). Three iterations were required to reach the final solution. Out of 94 initial missing is-a relations 37 were repaired by repairing actions which add new knowledge to the ontology while 57 were repaired using only the missing is-a relation itself. There were no derivable

	It1	It2	It3
Missing	94	101	101
Repaired by itself	57	98	101
Repaired using new knowledge	37	3	0
New relations	44	3	0

	It1	It2	It3
Missing	58	55	54
Repaired by itself	49	50	54
Repaired using new knowledge	9	5	0
New relations	6	4	0

(a) Results for debugging AMA - Mouse Anatomy ontology.   (b) Results for debugging NCI-A - Human Anatomy ontology.

Fig. 4. OAEI experiments

relations. In total 44 new and non-redundant relations were added to the ontology in the first iteration. Out of 37 relations which were repaired by adding new relations, 22 had more than 1 non-redundant relation in the repairing action. For example, the missing is-a relation wrist joint $\sqsubseteq$ joint is repaired by a repairing action {limb joint $\sqsubseteq$ joint, wrist joint $\sqsubseteq$ synovial joint}.

The set of missing is-a relations in the second iteration contains 101 relations, i.e. 57 relations which were repaired by adding the missing is-a relation itself and 44 newly added relations. In this iteration, 3 is-a relations were repaired by adding new knowledge to the ontology. All 3 of these is-a relations are is-a relations which were added in the previous iteration. For example, is-a relation wrist joint $\sqsubseteq$ synovial joint is repaired by a repairing action {wrist joint $\sqsubseteq$ hand joint} which is possible given that the is-a relation metacarpo-phalangeal joint $\sqsubseteq$ joint from the initial set of missing is-a relations was repaired by a repairing action {hand joint $\sqsubseteq$ synovial joint, limb joint $\sqsubseteq$ joint} in the first iteration. Finally, the set of missing is-a relations containing 101 is-a relations in the third iteration is also the solution for the initial set of missing is-a relations given that no new relations were added in the third iteration.

NCI – Human Anatomy. The initial set of missing is-a relations contained 58 relations for the NCI-A ontology. Out of these 58 relations in the first iteration 9 were repaired by adding relations which introduce new knowledge to the ontology. In total 6 new is-a relations were added and 4 missing is-a relations were derivable.

In the second iteration, 5 out of 55 is-a relations were repaired by adding new relations while repairing actions for the 50 other is-a relations were unchanged. All 5 is-a relations which were repaired by adding new relations to the ontology are is-a relations which were repaired by repairing actions containing only the missing is-a relation from the first iteration. This exemplifies why it is beneficial to consider already repaired is-a relations in subsequent iterations as Source and Target sets for some missing is-a relations can change and more informative solutions might be identified. The input to the third iteration is a set of 54 is-a relations and given that no changes were made, these relations are the final solution.

5.2   Case 2 Experiment – Biotop

This experiment relates to Case 2. In this experiment we used the Biotop ontology from the 2013 OWL Reasoner Evaluation Workshop dataset containing 280 concepts

	It1	It2	It3	It4
Missing	47	41	42	41
Repaired by itself	19	31	38	41
Repaired using new knowledge	28	10	4	0
New relations	26(3)	11	3(1)	0

Fig. 5. Results for debugging the Biotop ontology

and 42 object properties. For the set of missing is-a relations we randomly selected 47 is-a relations. Then the ontology was modified by removing is-a relations which would make the selected is-a relations derivable. The unmodified ontology was used as domain knowledge in the experiment. The results for debugging Biotop ontology are presented in Figure 5.

The debugging process took 4 iterations. In the first iteration 28 relations were repaired by adding new relations. In total 26 new relations were added in the first iteration using axioms containing $\exists$ expressions. For example, for missing is-a relation GreatApe $\sqsubseteq$ Primate we have a repairing action {FamilyHominidaeQuality $\sqsubseteq$ OrderPrimatesQuality} given that the ontology contains axioms GreatApe $\sqsubseteq$ $\exists$hasInherence.-FamilyHominidaeQuality and $\exists$hasInherence.OrderPrimatesQuality $\sqsubseteq$ Primate.

The input to the second iteration contained 41 non-redundant is-a relations (4 redundant is-a relations were removed from the solution in iteration 1). In total 10 is-a relations were repaired by adding new is-a relations. Out of these 10 repaired is-a relations, 5 are relations from the initial set of missing is-a relations while the other 5 are relations which were added in the first iteration. For example, is-a relation Atom $\sqsubseteq$ Entity from the initial set of missing relations can be repaired with {Atom $\sqsubseteq$ MaterialEntity} given that MaterialEntity $\sqsubseteq$ Entity was added in the previous iteration.

In the third iteration, the input contained 42 is-a relations. In total 4 is-a relations (3 from the initial set of missing is-a relations and 1 from iteration 1) were repaired by adding 3 new relations. Out of the 3 new relations 1 is acquired using axioms containing $\exists$ expressions. Finally, in the fourth iteration no new relations were added and the system outputs the solution.

5.3   Lessons Learned

The experiments have shown the usefulness of our approach. In each of the cases, whether missing is-a relations were identified, or whether we investigated existing is-a relations, our approach identified new information to be added to the ontologies.

The experiments have also shown that the iterative approach to repairing missing is-a relations is beneficial as in all our experiments additional relations were added to the ontology in subsequent iterations. Running the system on already repaired is-a relations gives the opportunity to identify new repairing actions which introduce new knowledge to the ontology. An example of this is found in the BioTop experiment where is-a relations from the initial set of missing is-a relations were repaired by more informative solutions in the third iteration.

Currently, the system removes redundant is-a relations from a solution after every iteration. This step is crucial for producing skyline optimal solutions. However, in situations where an is-a relation is repaired by a relation acquired from the axioms containing ∃ expressions it might be advantageous to keep also the missing is-a relation in subsequent iterations even though it is redundant. The reason for this is that the Source set and the Target set for the missing is-a relation might get updated in later iterations and therefore new repairing actions might be identified. One way to solve this is to make it possible in the system to show these missing is-a relations with their Source and Target sets but not to include them in the solution unless they are repaired using new knowledge. For example, let us assume that the missing is-a relation Human $\sqsubseteq$ Primate was repaired in one iteration by a repairing action {Human $\sqsubseteq$ Primate, SpeciesHomoSapiensQuality $\sqsubseteq$ OrderPrimatesQuality} in which case the second relation was found using ∃. In the next iteration the relation GreatApe $\sqsubseteq$ Primate was added to the ontology. If the system removed redundant relation Human $\sqsubseteq$ Primate then relation Human $\sqsubseteq$ GreatApe would not be detected as a possible repairing action for Human $\sqsubseteq$ Primate.

6 Related Work

There is not much work on the *completing of missing is-a structure*. In [26,25] this was addressed in the setting of taxonomies where the problem as well as some preference criteria were defined. Further, an algorithm was given and an implemented system was proposed. We note that the algorithm presented in this paper can be restricted to taxonomies and in that case finds more informative solutions than [26]. A later version of the [26] system, presented in [24], also deals with semantic defects, and was used for debugging ontologies related to a project for the Swedish National Food Agency [15]. An extension dealing with both ontology debugging and ontology alignment is described in [16]. In [23] the problem was formalized as an abduction problem and an algorithm was given for finding solutions for $\mathcal{ALC}$ acyclic terminologies. In [28] we extended the previous formalization by formalizing the role of the domain expert as well as by introducing preference criteria for the solutions to the problem. There is no other work yet on *GTAP*. There is some work on TBox abduction. [14] proposes an automata-based approach to TBox abduction in $\mathcal{EL}$. It is based on a reduction to the axiom pinpointing problem which is then solved with automata-based methods.

Further, there is work that addresses *related topics* but not directly the problem that is addressed in this paper. There is much work on the *detection of missing (is-a) relations* in e.g. ontology learning [4] or evolution [12], using linguistic [13] and logical [6] patterns, or by using knowledge intrinsic to an ontology network [26,15]. As mentioned before, these approaches, in general, do not detect all missing is-a relations. There is also much work on a dual problem to the one addressed in this paper, i.e. the *debugging of semantic defects*. Most of the work on debugging semantic defects aims at identifying and removing logical contradictions from an ontology [11,31,20,19,10], from mappings between ontologies [29,32,17,30] or ontologies in a network [18,15].

Finally, there is also work on other *abductive reasoning problems in (simple) description logics* including concept abduction [5,2,7] and ABox abduction [8,22,3] as defined in [9].

7 Conclusions

In this paper we presented an approach for completing the is-a structure of $\mathcal{EL}$ ontologies. Many biomedical ontologies can be represented by $\mathcal{EL}$ or a small extension thereof. We have also presented an implemented system and evaluated our approach on three biomedical ontologies. The evaluation has shown the usefulness of the system as in all experiments new is-a relations have been identified.

There are a number of directions for future work. We will investigate approaches for more expressive representation languages as well as different preference criteria. Further, we want to investigate methods for dealing with inconsistency and incoherence as well as incompleteness.

Acknowledgments. We thank the Swedish Research Council (Vetenskapsrådet), the Swedish e-Science Research Centre (SeRC) and the Swedish National Graduate School in Computer Science for financial support.

References

1. Baader, F., Brandt, S., Lutz, C.: Pushing the $\mathcal{EL}$ envelope. In: 19th Int. Joint Conf. on Artificial Intelligence, pp. 364–369 (2005)
2. Bienvenu, M.: Complexity of abduction in the $\mathcal{EL}$ family of lightweight description logics. In: 11th Int. Conf. on Principles of Knowledge Representation and Reasoning, pp. 220–230 (2008)
3. Calvanese, D., Ortiz, M., Simkus, M., Stefanoni, G.: The complexity of explaining negative query answers in DL-Lite. In: 13th Int. Conf. on Principles of Knowledge Representation and Reasoning, pp. 583–587 (2012)
4. Cimiano, P., Buitelaar, P., Magnini, B.: Ontology Learning from Text: Methods, Evaluation and Applications. IOS Press (2005)
5. Colucci, S., Di Noia, T., Di Sciascio, E., Donini, F., Mongiello, M.: A uniform tableaux-based approach to concept abduction and contraction in $\mathcal{ALN}$. In: Int. Workshop on Description Logics, pp. 158–167 (2004)
6. Corcho, O., Roussey, C., Vilches, L.M., Pérez, I.: Pattern-based OWL ontology debugging guidelines. In: Workshop on Ontology Patterns, pp. 68–82 (2009)
7. Donini, F., Colucci, S., Di Noia, T., Sciasco, E.D.: A tableaux-based method for computing least common subsumers for expressive description logics. In: 21st Int. Joint Conf. on Artificial Intelligence, pp. 739–745 (2009)
8. Du, J., Qi, G., Shen, Y.-D., Pan, J.: Towards practical abox abduction in large OWL DL ontologies. In: 25th AAAI Conf. on Artificial Intelligence, pp. 1160–1165 (2011)
9. Elsenbroich, C., Kutz, O., Sattler, U.: A case for abductive reasoning over ontologies. In: OWL: Experiences and Directions (2006)
10. Flouris, G., Manakanatas, D., Kondylakis, H., Plexousakis, D., Antoniou, G.: Ontology Change: Classification and Survey. Knowledge Engineering Review 23(2), 117–152 (2008)
11. Haase, P., Stojanovic, L.: Consistent Evolution of OWL Ontologies. In: Gómez-Pérez, A., Euzenat, J. (eds.) ESWC 2005. LNCS, vol. 3532, pp. 182–197. Springer, Heidelberg (2005)
12. Hartung, M., Terwilliger, J., Rahm, E.: Recent advances in schema and ontology evolution. In: Schema Matching and Mapping, pp. 149–190 (2011)
13. Hearst, M.: Automatic acquisition of hyponyms from large text corpora. In: 14th Int. Conf. on Computational Linguistics, pp. 539–545 (1992)

14. Hubauer, T., Lamparter, S., Pirker, M.: Automata-based abduction for tractable diagnosis. In: Int. Workshop on Description Logics, pp. 360–371 (2010)

15. Ivanova, V., Bergman, J.L., Hammerling, U., Lambrix, P.: Debugging taxonomies and their alignments: the ToxOntology - MeSH use case. In: 1st Int. Workshop on Debugging Ontologies and Ontology Mappings, pp. 25–36 (2012)

16. Ivanova, V., Lambrix, P.: A unified approach for aligning taxonomies and debugging taxonomies and their alignments. In: Cimiano, P., Corcho, O., Presutti, V., Hollink, L., Rudolph, S. (eds.) ESWC 2013. LNCS, vol. 7882, pp. 1–15. Springer, Heidelberg (2013)

17. Ji, Q., Haase, P., Qi, G., Hitzler, P., Stadtmüller, S.: RaDON — repair and diagnosis in ontology networks. In: Aroyo, L., Traverso, P., Ciravegna, F., Cimiano, P., Heath, T., Hyvönen, E., Mizoguchi, R., Oren, E., Sabou, M., Simperl, E. (eds.) ESWC 2009. LNCS, vol. 5554, pp. 863–867. Springer, Heidelberg (2009)

18. Jiménez-Ruiz, E., Cuenca Grau, B., Horrocks, I., Berlanga, R.: Ontology integration using mappings: Towards getting the right logical consequences. In: Aroyo, L., Traverso, P., Ciravegna, F., Cimiano, P., Heath, T., Hyvönen, E., Mizoguchi, R., Oren, E., Sabou, M., Simperl, E. (eds.) ESWC 2009. LNCS, vol. 5554, pp. 173–187. Springer, Heidelberg (2009)

19. Kalyanpur, A., Parsia, B., Sirin, E., Cuenca-Grau, B.: Repairing unsatisfiable concepts in OWL ontologies. In: Sure, Y., Domingue, J. (eds.) ESWC 2006. LNCS, vol. 4011, pp. 170–184. Springer, Heidelberg (2006)

20. Kalyanpur, A., Parsia, B., Sirin, E., Hendler, J.: Debugging Unsatisfiable Classes in OWL Ontologies. J. of Web Semantics 3(4), 268–293 (2006)

21. Kazakov, Y., Krötzsch, M., Simančík, F.: Concurrent classification of $\mathcal{EL}$ ontologies. In: Aroyo, L., Welty, C., Alani, H., Taylor, J., Bernstein, A., Kagal, L., Noy, N., Blomqvist, E. (eds.) ISWC 2011, Part I. LNCS, vol. 7031, pp. 305–320. Springer, Heidelberg (2011)

22. Klarman, S., Endriss, U., Schlobach, S.: Abox abduction in the description logic $\mathcal{ALC}$. J. of Automated Reasoning 46, 43–80 (2011)

23. Lambrix, P., Dragisic, Z., Ivanova, V.: Get my pizza right: Repairing missing is-a relations in $\mathcal{ALC}$ ontologies. In: Takeda, H., Qu, Y., Mizoguchi, R., Kitamura, Y. (eds.) JIST 2012. LNCS, vol. 7774, pp. 17–32. Springer, Heidelberg (2013)

24. Lambrix, P., Ivanova, V.: A unified approach for debugging is-a structure and mappings in networked taxonomies. J. of Biomedical Semantics 4, 10 (2013)

25. Lambrix, P., Liu, Q.: Debugging the missing is-a structure within taxonomies networked by partial reference alignments. Data & Knowledge Engineering 86, 179–205 (2013)

26. Lambrix, P., Liu, Q., Tan, H.: Repairing the Missing is-a Structure of Ontologies. In: Gómez-Pérez, A., Yu, Y., Ding, Y. (eds.) ASWC 2009. LNCS, vol. 5926, pp. 76–90. Springer, Heidelberg (2009)

27. Lambrix, P., Strömbäck, L., Tan, H.: Information Integration in Bioinformatics with Ontologies and Standards (chapter 8). In: Bry, F., Małuszyński, J. (eds.) Semantic Techniques for the Web. LNCS, vol. 5500, pp. 343–376. Springer, Heidelberg (2009)

28. Lambrix, P., Wei-Kleiner, F., Dragisic, Z., Ivanova, V.: Repairing missing is-a structure in ontologies is an abductive reasoning problem. In: 2nd Int. Workshop on Debugging Ontologies and Ontology Mappings, pp. 33–44 (2013)

29. Meilicke, C., Stuckenschmidt, H., Tamilin, A.: Repairing Ontology Mappings. In: 22nd Nat. Conf. on Artificial Intelligence, pp. 1408–1413 (2007)

30. Qi, G., Ji, Q., Haase, P.: A conflict-based operator for mapping revision. In: Bernstein, A., Karger, D.R., Heath, T., Feigenbaum, L., Maynard, D., Motta, E., Thirunarayan, K. (eds.) ISWC 2009. LNCS, vol. 5823, pp. 521–536. Springer, Heidelberg (2009)

31. Schlobach, S.: Debugging and Semantic Clarification by Pinpointing. In: Gómez-Pérez, A., Euzenat, J. (eds.) ESWC 2005. LNCS, vol. 3532, pp. 226–240. Springer, Heidelberg (2005)

32. Wang, P., Xu, B.: Debugging ontology mappings: a static approach. Computing and Informatics 27, 21–36 (2008)

Annotation-Based Feature Extraction
from Sets of SBML Models

Rebekka Alm[1,2], Dagmar Waltemath[3], Olaf Wolkenauer[3,4], and Ron Henkel[3]

[1] Dept. of Multimedia Communication, University of Rostock, Germany
[2] Fraunhofer Institute for Computer Graphics Rostock, Germany
rebekka.alm@igd-r.fraunhofer.de
[3] Dept. of Systems Biology and Bioinformatics, University of Rostock, Germany
{dagmar.waltemath|olaf.wolkenhauer|ron.henkel}@uni-rostock.de
[4] Stellenbosch Institute for Advanced Study (STIAS), Wallenberg Research Centre
at Stellenbosch University, Stellenbosh, South Africa

Abstract. Model repositories such as BioModels Database provide computational models of biological systems for the scientific community. These models contain rich semantic annotations that link model entities to concepts in well-established bio-ontologies such as Gene Ontology. Consequently, thematically similar models are likely to share similar annotations. Based on this assumption, we argue that semantic annotations are a suitable tool to characterize sets of models. These characteristics can then help to classify models, to identify additional features for model retrieval tasks, or to enable the comparison of sets of models. In this paper, we present four methods for annotation-based feature extraction from model sets. All methods have been used with four different model sets in SBML format and taken from BioModels Database. To characterize each of these sets, we analyzed and extracted concepts from three frequently used ontologies for SBML models, namely Gene Ontology, ChEBI and SBO. We find that three of the four tested methods are suitable to determine characteristic features for model sets. The selected features vary depending on the underlying model set, and they are also specific to the chosen model set. We show that the identified features map on concepts that are higher up in the hierarchy of the ontologies than the concepts used for model annotations. Our analysis also reveals that the information content of concepts in ontologies and their usage for model annotation do not correlate.

1 Introduction

Thanks to successful standardization efforts in Systems Biology [1], modelers today have access to high-quality, curated models in standard formats. The Systems Biology Markup Language (SBML) [2] is an XML-based standard format to encode models as interactions between biological entities. The emerging networks are furthermore enriched with semantic annotations [3] which link model parts to external knowledge in domain-specific ontologies (bio-ontologies, [4]). Many SBML models live in open model repositories such as BioModels Database [5].

H. Galhardas and E. Rahm (Eds.): DILS 2014, LNBI 8574, pp. 81–95, 2014.

The repository offers basic functionality for model management, including model collection, annotation, search, version control, data visualization etc.

BioModels Database implements a native, SQL-based search [5]. An alternative search, implemented in the BioModels Demo branch[1], is the *ranked model retrieval* [6]. Here, models and their annotations are mapped on pre-defined model features (e. g., model organism, author, biological entity), leading to a characteristic term vector for each model. The properties of this vector are numeric values mostly describing term frequency and inverse document frequency (TF-IDF) [7]. The ranking is determined by the comparison of search terms (i. e. provided keywords) with the extracted characteristic term vector per model. One drawback of this method is that standard Information Retrieval (IR) methods do not take into consideration the information hidden in semantic annotations. The major problem, however, is that current approaches only compare a set of keywords against an indexed corpus of documents. The set of keywords can either be user input, or a document transformed into a set of keywords. In both cases it is impossible to compare a *set* of documents with the corpus or with another set of documents, respectively. This is because it is problematic to identify suitable characteristics of arbitrary sets of models. For example, a standard search for "cell cycle" models will retrieve all models in the corpus that are relevant to the term "cell cycle". The result when querying BioModels Database is a large set of models. If relevant features for this set were pre-determined computationally for the corpus of interest, then the search results would be more specific to the topic of cell cycle. In other words, the possibility to identify characteristic features of a corpus at search time enables systems to only retrieve relevant models for a given research area.

In this paper we present four methods for annotation-based feature extraction from arbitrary sets of models. These methods rely on combinations of existing approaches for feature extractions. As an example, we compare the characteristic features of a set of cell cycle models to the features of arbitrary sets of models. Concepts were extracted from three major bio-ontologies used in models (GO, ChEBI, SBO). Our methods contribute to the determination of similarity between sets of models. They also provide statistics on the use of ontology terms in models, and on the relation between ontology terms and models.

2   Background

2.1   Bio-ontologies

SBML is an XML format. It uses an RDF scheme to add semantic annotations to model parts [8]. Among the ontologies that are used to enrich SBML models, we chose here the following three ontologies, which we believe are the most relevant in model annotation: an ontology of gene and gene product attributes, the *Gene Ontology* (GO) [9]; an ontology of chemical entities, the *Chemical Entities in*

---

[1] http://www.ebi.ac.uk/biomodels-demo/

BIology (ChEBI) [10]; and an ontology for modeling in biology, the *Systems Biology Ontology* (SBO) [3].

The GO is proposed and maintained by the Gene Ontology Consortium. It aims at standardizing the representation of gene and gene product attributes across species and databases by a structured, precisely defined, common, controlled vocabulary. GO covers three domains. Terms within each domain are linked by `is-a` and `part-of` relationships. Additionally, each concept is linked to other kinds of information, including many gene and protein keyword databases.

ChEBI is an ontology of chemical entities of biological interest. All database entries are `is_a` linked within the ontology. Chemical classifications of ChEBI are aligned with the classification of chemical processes in the GO, and the majority of chemical processes in GO are defined in terms of the ChEBI entities that participate in them.

The SBO provides a set of controlled vocabularies of terms commonly used in Systems Biology. It consists of seven orthogonal branches. Terms within each branch are linked by standard `is_a` relationships. Formal ties to SBO have been developed for several representation formats in Systems Biology. SBML elements[2], for example, carry an optional `sboTerm` attribute, which allows for a precise definition of the meaning of encoded model entities and their relationships.

2.2 Feature Extraction from Ontologies

To identify annotation-based characteristics of models, we first reviewed existing methods for feature extraction from ontologies and tree structures. We found the following suitable for our purposes.

Document Frequency. is a text classification metric. It describes the number of documents in which a term occurs [11,12]. It is used to reduce a vocabulary by removing too rare or too common words. Common words may be removed, because they are not discriminating for any particular class. Rare words may be eliminated because they are considered non-informative for category prediction and not influential in global performance. With respect to bio-ontologies, we keep common concepts but remove rarely used concepts during the feature extraction process.

Cluster Analysis. approaches of hierarchical clustering [13] can be applied to our feature extraction task. The top-down approach starts with a cluster containing all concepts and splits this cluster into smaller groups. The bottom-up approach starts with clusters only containing one concept. Those clusters are merged to larger clusters. Usually the path length between the concepts, the depth of the concepts, and the local semantic density determine the distance between ontology concepts [14]. For one bio-ontology at a time, we group concepts, i. e. terms in the ontology, based on their distance in the ontology graph.

---

[2] Since Level 2 Version 2.

Information Content. is proposed as another approach to determine similarity between concepts in ontologies [15,16]: The more information two concepts have in common, the more similar they are. The information content of a concepts is dependent on the concepts's probability. The probability $p(c)$ is calculated by the frequency $freq(c)$ of the concept c and the count N of all concepts of the ontology. It is formally defined by Resnik [15]:

$$p(c) = \frac{freq(c)}{N} \tag{1}$$

If all concepts in an ontology are subordinate to one item, then this item has the greatest probability of 1, because its classification always applies. However, the smaller the probability of a concept is, the higher is its information content. The information content can be calculated by the negative logarithm of the likelihood:

$$IC(c) = -\log_2 p(c) \tag{2}$$

In order to determine the common information content of two concepts, one considers the deepest element that classifies both concepts together. The information content of this element is the degree of mutual information content.

Inter-ontology Links. have been considered by Trißl et al. [17]. They address the problem of overgeneralization when using parent concepts as representatives for their child concepts. The challenge of feature extraction in ontologies is to find summarizing features that do not generalize too strongly. Concepts further up in the ontology are less specific than concepts further down in the ontology and thus have less "information content". Counting the number of references of a concept and its successor concepts would rank the general concept always highest, as it has more references. The counting approach does not consider the loss of specificity when moving up the ontology. Trißl et al. propose a similarity-based scoring function where a general concept must be supported by more references to yield a good score of representativeness.

3   Implementation

As a proof of concept, we implemented the four different methods described in Section 4 in a prototype application, using four different test sets.

3.1   Prototype

The prototype implementation incorporates two major technologies. First, ontologies are imported using the OWL API[3] and the JFact[4] reasoner. The Web Ontology Language (OWL) is a specification of the World Wide Web Consortium (W3C) to create, publish and to distribute ontologies based on a formal description language [18]. Most bio-ontologies are available in OWL format.

---

[3] http://owlapi.sourceforge.net/
[4] http://jfact.sourceforge.net/

Second, all relevant information about the models and the ontologies is stored and linked in a graph database [19]. The graph database enables us to integrate the ontologies with the SBML models, which are best represented in a graph-like structure [20]. We imported the ontology concepts and their taxonomic relationships and counted the number of annotations referring from a model to a particular ontology concept. The storage approach is described in more detail in [21].

3.2 Test Sets

The test sets were built from SBML models in BioModels Database[5]. We only chose models from the curated branch of the repository, because these models are manually checked and fully annotated. The models were selected using our previously developed retrieval algorithm [6]. The first test set is a thematic set containing SBML encodings of published cell cycle models. We used the term "cell cycle" to retrieve a ranked list of relevant models. To exclude possible false positive search results we manually validated the retrieved models based on their reference publications, resulting in the 34 given models. Additionally, two random sets were assembled. Each set contains 34 models (Table 1).

Table 1. List of models contained in the four test sets: selection of published cell cycle models from BioModels Database; two random sets; and all curated models from Release 25 of BioModels Database.

Cell Cycle (*CC*)	Random Set 1 (*RS1*)	Random Set 2 (*RS2*)	BioModels Database (*BMDB*)
BIOMD0000000003	BIOMD0000000007	BIOMD0000000005	curated
BIOMD0000000005	BIOMD0000000015	BIOMD0000000010	branch
BIOMD0000000006	BIOMD0000000016	BIOMD0000000023	BioModels
BIOMD0000000007	BIOMD0000000029	BIOMD0000000048	Database
BIOMD0000000008	BIOMD0000000050	BIOMD0000000080	Release 25
BIOMD0000000056	BIOMD0000000061	BIOMD0000000081	(490 SBML files)
BIOMD0000000064	BIOMD0000000062	BIOMD0000000087	
BIOMD0000000069	BIOMD0000000075	BIOMD0000000105	
BIOMD0000000087	BIOMD0000000095	BIOMD0000000112	
BIOMD0000000107	BIOMD0000000107	BIOMD0000000118	
BIOMD0000000109	BIOMD0000000131	BIOMD0000000139	
BIOMD0000000110	BIOMD0000000173	BIOMD0000000141	
BIOMD0000000111	BIOMD0000000218	BIOMD0000000158	
BIOMD0000000144	BIOMD0000000225	BIOMD0000000168	
BIOMD0000000150	BIOMD0000000280	BIOMD0000000223	
BIOMD0000000168	BIOMD0000000290	BIOMD0000000254	
BIOMD0000000169	BIOMD0000000312	BIOMD0000000281	
BIOMD0000000181	BIOMD0000000314	BIOMD0000000282	
BIOMD0000000186	BIOMD0000000315	BIOMD0000000301	
BIOMD0000000187	BIOMD0000000324	BIOMD0000000313	
BIOMD0000000193	BIOMD0000000345	BIOMD0000000314	
BIOMD0000000194	BIOMD0000000361	BIOMD0000000315	
BIOMD0000000195	BIOMD0000000384	BIOMD0000000320	
BIOMD0000000196	BIOMD0000000391	BIOMD0000000335	
BIOMD0000000207	BIOMD0000000393	BIOMD0000000376	
BIOMD0000000208	BIOMD0000000425	BIOMD0000000391	
BIOMD0000000216	BIOMD0000000428	BIOMD0000000412	
BIOMD0000000228	BIOMD0000000433	BIOMD0000000418	
BIOMD0000000242	BIOMD0000000437	BIOMD0000000426	
BIOMD0000000265	BIOMD0000000455	BIOMD0000000433	
BIOMD0000000297	BIOMD0000000046	BIOMD0000000076	
BIOMD0000000318	BIOMD0000000117	BIOMD0000000253	
BIOMD0000000370	BIOMD0000000449	BIOMD0000000260	
BIOMD0000000409	BIOMD0000000471	BIOMD0000000429	

---

[5] ftp://ftp.ebi.ac.uk/pub/databases/biomodels/releases/
2013-06-18/BioModels_Database-r25_pub-sbml_files.tar.bz2

4   Results

We argued in the introduction that thematically similar models share similar annotations, and that it is possible to extract characteristic features from semantic annotations, both for specialized sets of models and for arbitrary ones. The following subsections describe four methods that identify characteristic features, based on the aforementioned feature extraction methods (Section 4.1); discuss their applicability to feature extraction from models (Section 4.2); show the distribution of model annotations (Section 4.3); and discuss the application of two methods to the test sets (Section 4.4). We conclude that it is indeed possible to identify characteristic features which then help in tasks such as model retrieval, comparison and clustering.

4.1   Methods for Feature Extractions from Bio-Models

The goal for all feature extraction approaches was to identify a predefined number of features for all sets of models shown in Table 1. All methods incorporate the ontology structure to group the concepts within the ontology. Parent concepts represent the group containing their child concepts. Consequently, the developed methods are only applicable to taxonomy-shaped ontologies. Method 1 depends only on the chosen ontology, but not on the input set of models. All other methods additionally consider the annotations in the given set of models.

Method 1. is a top-down clustering. To decide on the suitability of a concept for characterization, the probability p of each concept in the ontology is determined, following Resnik's definition (Equation 1). The frequency $freq(c)$ is in our context the number of all concepts that are summarized by a parent concept c.

Method 2. is a top-down clustering that considers both the ontology structure and the annotations used in models of the given set. Consequently, the real distribution of references to ontology concepts used in models is regarded. Selected features depend on the given set of models. For each concept in the ontology, we count the number of annotations that refer to it. We call this number entity frequency. Additionally, we store the sum of a concept's entity frequency and its descendants' entity frequencies as aggregated entity frequency EF. All concepts with $EF > 0$ provide the basis for feature extraction. Method 2 re-uses the algorithm of Method 1. The algorithm is adjusted to the dynamic setting by using the entity frequency metric instead of the probability $p(c)$. To better compare the balance of the branches, we will normalize EF as entity probability $ep(c)$:

$$ep(c) = \frac{EF(c)}{EF(root)} \tag{3}$$

Method 3. is a bottom-up clustering relying on the same input as Method 2. It also uses the entity probability $ep(c)$ but begins with the individual concepts, which are gradually merged to form greater clusters. Starting from the concepts farthest away from the root we try to merge children and parents into groups that are represented by the parent concept. We continue to merge concepts and groups until we have the predefined number of groups or until we reach the root. A group should not be represented by the root-concept for obvious reasons. If in the end there are too many groups left and no reasonable possibility to merge them anymore, the groups with a higher value of the aggregated entity frequency EF are preferred over the groups with less occurrences.

Method 4. is a bottom-up clustering that addresses the problem of overgeneralization. It uses an adaptation of the scoring function as described in [17]:

$$Score_T(c) = IC(c) \cdot EF(c) \qquad (4)$$

The $Score_T(c)$ for a grouping represented by the concept c considers the information content and the aggregated entity frequency $EF(c)$. The information content $IC(c)$ is calculated depending on the probability (see Equations 1 and 2). A group is formed by merging concepts with the ancestor that reaches the highest possible score.

4.2 Applicability to Feature Extraction from SBML Models

We tested the applicability of all described methods to the problem of feature extraction from sets of SBML models. Method 1 calculates the probability to hit a certain node in an ontology with a model entity. It condenses a given ontology to a defined number of features, based on the probability of a concept in the ontology only. Method 1 thus does not depend on model annotation, i.e. it does not depend on the actual ontology concepts that are referenced in the model set. Consequently, it does not adapt to the specifics of the corpus under study. Therefore, Method 1 is only suitable to provide a static set of features, solely based on the underlying ontology. We thus dismissed Method 1 for the problem of finding characteristics for arbitrary model sets. However, we find that Method 1 can give us an idea of the distribution of concepts in bio-ontologies, as shown in Section 4.3. Method 2 and Method 3 rely on entity probabilities. Our evaluations show that Method 2 (top-down) and Method 3 (bottom-up) produce almost identical results. The direction is only relevant in the rare constellation that two concepts are subsumed to the same score. We thus consider Method 2 for the following evaluations. Method 4 is a dynamic approach that calculates the score value by entity frequency and information content. Because of the unique scoring and the absence of splits, Method 4 generally finds a fewer number of features than the prior methods. However, the method selects specific features (further down in the ontology tree) that are still representative for the model sets. In summary, all four methods work and provide new insights.

We consider Method 2 and Method 4 most suitable for our application scenario.

4.3   Distribution of SBO Concepts in SBML Models

Using Method 1, it is possible to compare the distributions of concepts in a bio-ontology (here: SBO) with the frequency of annotations as they occur in all models from BioModels Database. Figure 1 (top) shows the unequal distributions of concepts in SBO across the seven top-level branches. The model annotations linking into SBO are also unbalanced, but differently (Figure 1, bottom). For example, the branch "physical entity representation" contains only 10% of SBO concepts, but 47% of the model annotations link to that branch.

Due to the unbalanced nature of SBO, we expect that the characteristic features follow the distribution of the model annotations as seen in the lower part of the figure. Section 4.4 discusses this assumption.

We also investigated for each model annotation at which depth the linked concepts occur in the ontology tree. This knowledge helps us to decide on how specific a model annotation is. Figure 2 shows the distribution for model annotations using ChEBI, GO and SBO. Here we plotted the distribution of annotations for the *CC* and the *BMDB* sets. As one would expect, both test sets show normal distributions. Interestingly, the number of annotations in the *CC* set that refer to ChEBI is less than 1% compared to the number of annotations in the *BMDB* set. This information helps us later on in Section 4.4 to decide on the value of the extracted features.

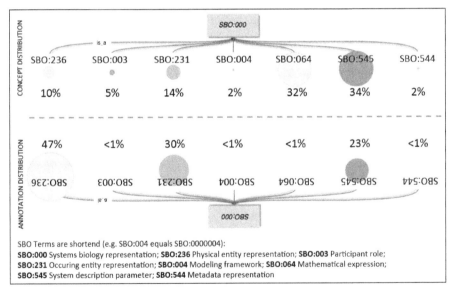

Fig. 1. Overview of the concept distribution in the seven branches of the Systems Biology Ontology (SBO). The size of the colored circles visualizes the number of concepts summarized by each branch. The bottom mirrored image visualizes the distribution of annotations from all models in the BioModels Database test set (BMDB). Figure adapted from [3].

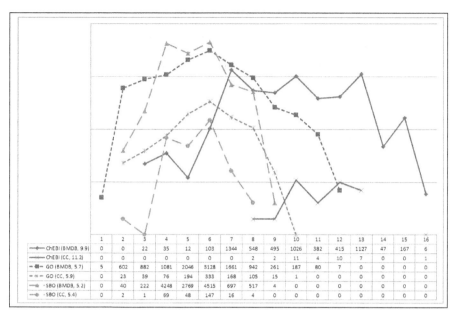

	1	2	3	4	5	6	7	8	9	10	11	12	13	14	15	16
ChEBI (BMDB, 9.9)	0	0	22	35	12	103	1344	548	495	1026	382	415	1127	47	167	6
ChEBI (CC, 11.2)	0	0	0	0	0	0	0	2	2	11	4	10	7	0	0	1
GO (BMDB, 5.7)	5	602	882	1081	2046	3128	1661	942	261	187	80	7	0	0	0	0
GO (CC, 5.9)	0	23	59	76	194	333	168	105	15	1	0	0	0	0	0	0
SBO (BMDB, 5.2)	0	40	222	4248	2769	4515	697	517	4	0	0	0	0	0	0	0
SBO (CC, 5.4)	0	2	1	69	48	147	16	4	0	0	0	0	0	0	0	0

Fig. 2. Distribution of annotation depth. Overview of the distribution of annotated model entities in relation to the depth of the annotation. The x-axis shows the depth of the annotated concepts in the corresponding ontology, the y-axis shows the number of annotated entities on a logarithmic scale (exact values are stated at the bottom of the figure). The figure legend states the ontology name, the model set (Table 1) and the average depth.

4.4   Feature Extraction from Arbitrary Model Sets

We hypothesis that the vast property space of a set of models can be condensed into a smaller, but still descriptive, number of features. To establish such "characteristic features", we collect the models' annotations and analyze the semantics behind the linked ontology terms. Apart from annotations, many other characteristics could also be incorporated when describing an SBML model, such as properties of the reaction networks or entity names and entity values [22]. However, we focus here on the semantics behind the model elements because we believe that this information will be most influential for the similarity. In BioModels Database, models carry between three and 800 annotations, with an average of 71 annotations per model [19]. As all our methods require setting a maximum number of features, we asked the question: "How many characteristic features are necessary to describe a model set?". Here we follow the Pareto-principle[6] and test our methods for upper limits of five and 15 features. The resulting sets of features for all feature extraction algorithms, models, and ontologies are shown in Table 2.

---

[6] 80/20 rule http://en.wikipedia.org/wiki/Pareto_principle

Table 2. Extracted features for different test sets, methods and feature size. The upper Table shows a maximum of five features, the bottom Table 15 features, respectively. IDs are shortened (e. g. SBO:0000064 is represented by 064) and ordered ascending. The average depth (*avg*) of features per ontology is emphasized for the CC and BMDB test sets.

5 Features	Method 2				Method 4			
	CC	RS1	RS2	BMDB	CC	RS1	RS2	BMDB
ChEBI	33285	24870	24870	24870	22563	22563	26816	24870
	33302	33302	33302	33302	33608	26082	33695	26082
	33304	33304	33304	33304	33694	33241	47019	33241
	35701	33582	33582	33582	37096	33695	61120	33695
	36357	36357	36357	36357	37787	61120	63367	61120
avg depth	5.4			4.2	7.2			5.4
GO	8152	3674	3674	3674	22411	3674	3674	3674
	9987	8152	5575	8152	30163	5575	9987	5575
	44699	9987	8152	9987	51726	6810	9987	9987
	65007	44699	9987	44699	65009	9987	43170	43170
	71840	51234	44699	65007	71822	43170	71822	71822
avg depth	2			1.8	4.4			2.6
SBO	003	064	231	003	009	009	009	003
	236	231	245	064	231	064	167	009
	374	240	247	231	252	176	240	064
	375	241	291	236	336	252		167
	545	545	545	545				240
avg depth	2.4			2	4			3

15 Features	Method 2				Method 4			
	CC	RS1	RS2	BMDB	CC	RS1	RS2	BMDB
ChEBI	16646	18059	18059	18059	22563	22563	24875	24835
	24651	24835	24835	24835	33608	24835	25107	24870
	25367	24870	24870	24870	33694	25741	26816	26082
	25699	25367	25367	25367	37096	26082	33252	33241
	25741	25806	26082	26082	37787	33241	33620	33259
	26082	26082	33259	33241		33252	33636	33636
	33241	26835	33304	33259		33259	33695	33695
	33839	33241	33581	33285		33608	35155	35155
	35701	33259	33674	33304		33695	35569	35569
	36358	33285	33839	33674		35701	47019	35701
	36606	33674	35701	33839		61120	61120	47019
	51143	33694	37577	35701		63367	63161	61120
	63161	35701	50906	50906		64709	63367	63161
	63299	51143	51143	51143				63367
	64709	64709	64709	64709				64709
avg depth	5.9			4.8	7.2			6.3
GO	3674	3674	3674	3674	216	3674	3674	3674
	5575	5575	5575	5575	4693	5575	5834	5575
	6807	6807	6807	8152	5575	6810	6826	9987
	9056	9056	9056	9987	22411	9987	8943	43170
	9058	9058	9058	32501	30163	16088	9987	71822
	40007	44237	32501	32502	32268	43170	22607	
	44237	44238	44237	40007	45750	45750	43170	
	44238	44699	44238	44699	51726		71822	
	44699	44710	44699	48511	65009			
	50896	48511	44710	50896	71822			
	51234	50896	50896	51234				
	65007	51234	51234	51704				
	71704	65007	65007	65007				
	71840	71704	71704	71840				
		71840	71840					
avg depth	2.3			1.8	4.1			2.6
SBO	009	064	016	003	009	009	009	003
	177	177	017	064	231	064	167	009
	179	179	046	241	252	176	240	064
	180	180	153	245	336	252		167
	181	182	156	247				240
	182	185	231	253				
	205	205	241	285				
	245	241	245	290				
	253	247	247	291				
	290	250	253	374				
	291	253	290	375				
	308	285	291	405				
	342	290	308	409				
	360	377	360	412				
	374	545	380	545				
avg depth	4.6			3.3	4			3

Specificity of Selected Ontology Concepts. Table 2 shows the average depth of concepts in all three ontologies for all identified features in the *CC* and *BMDB* sets. Additionally, Figure 2 contains the average depth of annotation for the *CC* and *BMDB* sets before applying the feature extraction methods. The data confirms that the average depth of annotations decreases for Methods 2 and 4 (for all three ontologies and both model sets). This means that the selected concepts are higher up in the ontology, and thus more generic. This behavior is expected as the feature extraction process also involves generalization. However, the features extracted by Method 4 are more specific than the features extracted by Method 2. This is in accordance with the design of Method 4 to prevent over-generalization. Also, the average annotation depth for the *CC* set is higher than for the corresponding *BMDB* set. This supports our assumption that thematically similar models share more annotations, and consequently the extracted features are more specific. For example, the concepts that were selected from ChEBI by Method 2 with a maximum of 15 features for the *CC* set have an average annotation depth of 5.9. In contrast, the concepts that were selected for the *BMDB* set only have an average depth of 4.8. According to our obtained data we can say that Method 4, in general, provides features that correspond to deeper concepts in the ontology than the features obtained from Method 2. We can conclude from our test data that the depth of chosen concepts decreases with the increased randomness in the sets of models. This is not unexpected, as a broader data basis should not be characterizable by very specific ontology concepts. Rather, an arbitrary model set should cover many different semantic concepts, leading to more generic features beeing extracted. This behavior is also reflected in our data. In summary, both methods extract features that are specific to the model set. In addition, features extracted by Method 4 are more specific than those extracted by Method 2. Features selected for the *CC* set are more specific as the models share many annotations.

Distinctness of Feature Sets. Another important question is how distinct the obtained features are for our test sets. If the methods retrieved similar concepts for the four test sets, then the extracted features could not be regarded specific to the set of models. Consequently, we could not assume to be able to improve the comparison of model sets based on these features. We thus were interested in the overlap of concepts between the different characteristic features that we calculated from Method 2 and Method 4. Ideally, there is almost no overlap of features selected for the *CC* set with any other selected set, whereas an overlap between *BMDB* and the random sets can be expected. Our results are shown in Figure 3. A good result is achieved for Method 4 using 15 features and GO. Here, the cell cycle features have almost no overlap. The result achieved for Method 2 using 15 features and GO is not satisfiable. Here, the cell cycle features largely overlap with at least two other sets. However, the Venn diagrams, in general, confirm that both methods determine features that are specific to the model sets. They contain higher numbers of overlapping features at the intersection between arbitrary sets and very few overlapping features at the intersection between the

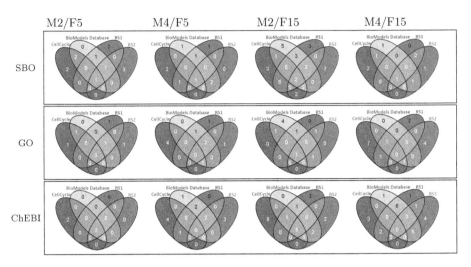

Fig. 3. Visualization of feature overlaps of the four test sets. Each diagram shows the overlap of the results of one ontology (SBO, GO or ChEBI), method (2 or 4) and number of features (5 or 15)

CC and the *BMDB* sets. This is particularly visible for the results obtained from Method 4.

Specificity of Extracted Features. We were also interested in how characteristic the sets of extracted features are for a given set of models. We first calculate the similarity of two concepts within the same ontology, as described by Li *et al.* [14]:

$$S(c_1, c_2) = e^{-\alpha l} \cdot \frac{e^{\beta h} - e^{-\beta h}}{e^{\beta h} + e^{-\beta h}} \tag{5}$$

The variable h is the depth of the least common subsumer of the concepts c_1 and c_2, and the variable l is the length of the shortest path between both concepts. Following [14], the parameters are set to $\alpha = 0.2$ and $\beta = 0.6$. We calculate this similarity value for each possible combination of features from two sets of models.

Afterwards we apply an adaptation of the Hungarian method [23] to the matrix resulting from the above calculations. The Hungarian method, a solution for the assignment problem, assigns pairs of features, so that a global maximum similarity is ensured. Based on this similarity of features we then calculate the total similarity of two sets of features, which corresponds to the similarity of the associated sets of models. The results are shown in Table 3. Desirable are low similarities for *BMDB vs CC* as well as *CC vs RS1*. As *CC* is a thematic set, its extracted features should differ from the features extracted from the *BMDB* and arbitrary model sets. Higher similarity is expected for *BMDB vs RS1*, as both sets represent a wide range of model topics. The results in Table 3 reflect our expectations. Particularly, the similarity values for Method 4 using 15 features

Table 3. Similarity between two model sets, calculated based on the similarity of their characteristic features

model sets	ontology	method/number of features			
		M2 F5	M4 F5	M2 F15	M4 F15
BMDB vs CC	ChEBI	0.82	0.57	0.75	0.20
	GO	0.80	0.40	0.71	0.30
	SBO	0.75	0.44	0.50	0.43
BMDB vs RS1	ChEBI	1.00	0.94	0.91	0.71
	GO	0.87	0.84	0.67	0.59
	SBO	0.75	0.65	0.63	0.65
CC vs RS1	ChEBI	0.82	0.63	0.77	0.29
	GO	0.67	0.25	0.90	0.36
	SBO	0.50	0.63	0.70	0.63

clearly distinguish the extracted features of two sets. Method 2 using 5 features still shows the desired result, but due to the limited number of features the selected ones are more general and thus not as distinguishable. Even though results of Method 2 show the expected behaviour, we conclude that the results of Method 4 are superior.

Distribution of SBO Concepts. Finally, we investigate the distribution of the selected SBO features for the *BMDB* set with respect to the SBO top level entries. As discussed earlier, Figure 1 shows a mismatch between available concepts and used concepts. We assume a similar distribution of concepts after applying our feature extraction methods. Indeed, after applying Method 4, the selected features show a distribution in SBO that is similar to the one in Figure 1: 66.6% SBO:236, 6.6% SBO:003, 13.3% SBO:231, 6.6% SBO:064, and 6.6% SBO:545 (see also Table 2, Method 4, SBO, 15 features).

5   Summary

This paper presents and discusses methods for the annotation-based extraction of characteristic features from sets of SBML models. The methods consider clustering and text classification techniques to extract characterizing features for sets of annotated computational models in biology. Annotation-based feature extraction enables the comparison of sets of models, as opposed to existing methods for model-to-keyword comparison, or model-to-model comparison.

We evaluated four different methods for feature extraction and conclude that Method 4 is the most suitable. This method considers both, the semantic annotations in a set of models, and the information content of the referenced ontologies. We showed that these features are specific and distinct. At the same time the features are not overgeneralized. We also showed how to assign a similarity value to sets of models, based on the similarity of the extracted features. In summary, our expectations have been met: A thematic set of models, for example cell cycle models, can computationally be distinguished from an arbitrary set of models.

Our methods are format agnostic and expandable. They can be adapted to other model representation formats such as CellML [24] or NeuroML [25]. Interestingly, these extensions enable a comparison between sets of models of arbitrary formats. It is also possible to incorporate further bio-ontologies, e. g. BRENDA [26]. For the near future, we plan to integrate Method 4 in our system for ranked model retrieval [6]. We wish to test the implications of feature extraction on model comparison and, in particular, model retrieval. We will also incorporate a larger set of ontologies into our system and ultimately in the process of feature extraction.

References

1. Le Novère, N., et al.: Meeting report from the first meetings of the Computational Modeling in Biology Network (COMBINE). Standards in Genomic Sciences 5(2), 230 (2011)
2. Hucka, M., et al.: The systems biology markup language (SBML): a medium for representation and exchange of biochemical network models. Bioinformatics 19(4), 524–531 (2003)
3. Courtot, M., et al.: Controlled vocabularies and semantics in systems biology. Molecular Systems Biology 7(1) (2011)
4. Robinson, P.N., Bauer, S.: Introduction to Bio-ontologies. Taylor & Francis, US (2011)
5. Li, C., et al.: BioModels Database: An enhanced, curated and annotated resource for published quantitative kinetic models. BMC Systems Biology 4(1), 92 (2010)
6. Henkel, R., et al.: Ranked retrieval of Computational Biology models. BMC Bioinformatics 11(1), 423 (2010)
7. Baeza-Yates, R., Ribeiro-Neto, B.: Modern Information Retrieval. ACM Press Books (1999)
8. Waltemath, D., et al.: SBML Level 3 Package Proposal: Annot. Nature Preceedings (2011), http://precedings.nature.com/documents/5610/version/1
9. Ashburner, M., et al.: Gene Ontology: tool for the unification of biology. Nature Genetics 25(1), 25–29 (2000)
10. Hastings, J., et al.: The ChEBI reference database and ontology for biologically relevant chemistry: enhancements for 2013. Nucleic Acids Res. 41, D456–D463 (2013)
11. Yang, Y., Pedersen, J.O.: A Comparative Study on Feature Selection in Text Categorization. In: Proceedings of the Fourteenth International Conference on Machine Learning, ICML 1997, San Francisco, CA, USA, pp. 412–420. Morgan Kaufmann Publishers Inc. (1997)
12. Forman, G.: An extensive empirical study of feature selection metrics for text classification. J. Mach. Learn. Res. 3, 1289–1305 (2003)
13. Hastie, T., Tibshirani, R., Friedman, J.: Hierarchical Clustering. In: The Elements of Statistical Learning, pp. 520–528. Springer (2009)
14. Li, Y., et al.: An approach for measuring semantic similarity between words using multiple information sources. IEEE Transactions on Knowledge and Data Engineering 15(4), 871–882 (2003)
15. Resnik, P.: Using information content to evaluate semantic similarity in a taxonomy. In: Proceedings of the 14th International Joint Conference on Artificial Intelligence, pp. 445–453 (1995)
16. Resnik, P.: Semantic similarity in a taxonomy: An information-based measure and its application to problems of ambiguity in natural language. Journal of Artificial Intelligence Research 11, 95–130 (1999)

17. Trißl, S., Hussels, P., Leser, U.: InterOnto – Ranking Inter-Ontology Links. In: Bodenreider, O., Rance, B. (eds.) DILS 2012. LNCS, vol. 7348, pp. 5–20. Springer, Heidelberg (2012)

18. McGuinness, D.L., et al.: Owl web ontology language overview. W3C Recommendation 10(2004-03) (2004)

19. Henkel, R., Wolkenhauer, O., Walthemath, D.: Combining computational models, semantic annotations, and associated simulation experiments in a graph database. Peer J. Preprints (2:e376v1) (2014)

20. Waltemath, D., et al.: Possibilities for Integrating Model-related Data in Computational Biology. In: CEUR Workshop Proceedings of the 9th International Conference on Data Integration in the Life Sciences (2013), http://www2.unb.ca/csas/data/ws/dils2013/

21. Henkel, R., et al.: Considerations of graph-based concepts to manage computational biology models and associated simulations. In: GI-Jahrestagung, pp. 1545–1551 (2012)

22. Waltemath, D., et al.: Das Sombi-Framework zum Ermitteln geeigneter Suchfunktionen für biologische Modelldatenbasen. Datenbank-Spektrum 11(1), 27–36 (2011)

23. Kuhn, H.W.: The hungarian method for the assignment problem. Naval Research Logistics Quarterly 2(1-2), 83–97 (1955)

24. Cuellar, A.A., et al.: An overview of CellML 1.1, a biological model description language. Simulation 79(12), 740–747 (2003)

25. Gleeson, P., et al.: NeuroML: a language for describing data driven models of neurons and networks with a high degree of biological detail. PLoS Computational Biology 6(6), e1000815 (2010)

26. Schomburg, I., et al.: BRENDA in 2013: integrated reactions, kinetic data, enzyme function data, improved disease classification: new options and contents in BRENDA. Nucleic Acids Research 41(D1), D764–D772 (2013)

REX – A Tool for Discovering Evolution Trends in Ontology Regions

Victor Christen[1], Anika Groß[1,2], and Michael Hartung[1,2]

[1] Department of Computer Science, Universität Leipzig, Germany
[2] Interdisciplinary Center for Bioinformatics, Universität Leipzig, Germany
mam08bfa@studserv.uni-leipzig.de,
{gross,hartung}@informatik.uni-leipzig.de

Abstract. A large number of life science ontologies has been developed to support different application scenarios such as gene annotation or functional analysis. The continuous accumulation of new insights and knowledge affects specific portions in ontologies and thus leads to their adaptation. Therefore, it is valuable to study which ontology parts have been extensively modified or remained unchanged. Users can monitor the evolution of an ontology to improve its further development or apply the knowledge in their applications. Here we present REX (Region Evolution Explorer) a web-based system for exploring the evolution of ontology parts (regions). REX provides an interactive and user-friendly interface to identify (un)stable regions in large life science ontologies and is available at http://www.izbi.de/rex.

Keywords: ontologies, ontology evolution, graph vizualisation.

1 Introduction and Background

In recent years ontologies have become increasingly important for annotating, sharing and analyzing data in the life sciences [1,8]. The heavy usage of ontologies leads to a steady modification of their content [7,9]. In particular, ontologies are adapted to incorporate new knowledge, eliminate initial design errors or achieve changed requirements. Tools like Protégé [16] support the development and change of ontologies. This process is usually distributed since especially large ontologies can not be maintained by single developers, such that collaborative work is performed [3,16]. Typically, the overall development of an ontology is coordinated by a project leader or consortium, and multiple developers contribute knowledge in their field of expertise.

Due to the ontology's size and complexity, the problem arises that coordinators, developers and users want to know whether specific parts (regions) of a large ontology have changed or not. For instance, if a user considers the anatomy part of the NCI Thesaurus (NCIT) [13] for annotating local data such as radiology pictures, she would like to know how this part has evolved recently, i.e., is the part unstable or stable. Unstable regions have been in the focus of development and underlay many modifications. By contrast, a stable region might be

H. Galhardas and E. Rahm (Eds.): DILS 2014, LNBI 8574, pp. 96–103, 2014.

already completed or was of low interest during recent ontology development. Project coordinators are interested in the evolution of different ontology parts (1) to see how work has progressed and (2) to detect potential for future development. Moreover ontology-based algorithms or applications might be affected by ontology changes. For instance, if results of a gene set enrichment analysis [15] are located in a strongly evolving ontology part, it should be re-done based on the newest ontology version to see how results change [2]. By contrast, results located within stable ontology parts are likely to remain unchanged.

Currently, life science ontologies can be accessed through platforms like Bio-Portal [10] and OBO Foundry [14]. Although it is possible to retrieve different versions of an ontology, such platforms rarely provide information about evolution, i.e., users have the problem to figure out how an ontology has evolved compared to their version in use. Recently, some web tools offer access to information about the evolution of the Gene Ontology (GO). GOChase [12] allows to study the history of individual GO concepts and Park et al. [11] propose graph-based visualization methods to view modified GO terms. In own previous work we designed the OnEX web application [6] for quantitative and concept-based evolution analyses in life science ontologies. Our tool CODEX [5] can be used to determine a diff between two ontology versions covering complex changes (e.g., concept merge or split). For a general overview on ontology and schema evolution including diff computation we refer to [7]. In summary, currently available tools lack the functionality to analyze and compare evolution in different ontology parts especially for large ontologies with several version releases. In own previous work [4] we already proposed an algorithm to detect (un)stable ontology regions for an arbitrary number of ontology versions. However, the algorithm is only applicable offline, i.e., the research community can not make use of it.

We therefore present the novel web application REX (Region Evolution Explorer) based on the region discovery algorithm [4]. REX can be used (1) to determine differently changing regions for periodically updated ontologies, and (2) to interactively explore the change intensity of those regions. REX provides a comparative trend analysis such that users and developers can monitor the long-term evolution for their regions of interest, e.g., to track the work or coordinate future development. REX is online available at `http://www.izbi.de/rex`.

2   Region Discovery Method

The region discovery method proposed in [4] enables the detection of changing and stable ontology regions. The basic idea is to compute change intensities for regions based on changes between several succeeding versions of an ontology within a specific time interval. The algorithm consists of four main steps: (1) change computation, (2) cost propagation, (3) cost transfer, and (4) region discovery. It first computes differences between two versions to determine changes. It then propagates change costs within the *is-a* hierarchy of the ontology and transfers these costs from the first to the last considered version. Based on computed change intensities we can discover differently evolving ontology regions. First, we briefly describe the method for two input versions O_{old} and O_{new}.

Table 1. Change operations and change cost model used in REX

	Change operation	Description	Change costs
Concepts	addC	addition of a new concept	1
	delC	deletion of a concept	2
Relationships	addR	addition of a new relationship	0.5/0.5
	delR	deletion of a relationship	1.0/1.0
Attributes	addA	addition of a new attribute	0.5
	delA	deletion of an attribute	0.5
	chgAttValue	modification / change of an attribute value	0.5

In general, ontology content can be added (addition), removed (deletion) or modified (update). Here we distinguish between the basic change operations for ontology concepts, their attributes and relationships between concepts listed in Table 1. Our region discovery method assigns so-called local costs $lc(c)$ to concepts to cover the impact of changes that directly influence a concept c (see change costs in Table 1). For instance, we can assign higher costs to deletions since they might have a higher impact on dependent applications than additions. Note, that the cost model can be adapted according to the application scenario. Additions are registered in the new version while deletions are covered in the old version. Moreover, the assignment depends on which ontology element has changed. Here we assign costs from changes on a concept or its attributes to the concept itself. Costs for relationships are split and assigned to the source and target concept of the relationship, respectively. The local costs are then propagated along *is-a* paths upwards in the ontology hierarchy to obtain aggregated costs. Due to multi-inheritance we may need to split costs during propagation. We therefore determine aggregated costs $ac(c)$ for a concept c as follows:

$$ac(c) = \sum_{c' \in children(c)} \frac{ac(c')}{|parents(c')|} + lc(c)$$

We thus ensure that the root concept(s) of the ontology contain the overall sum of all assigned local costs. Fig. 1 (left) shows an exemplary anatomy ontology with local and aggregated costs. For instance, the aggregated costs of 'organ' $(ac('organ') = 6)$ are computed based on the aggregated costs of its children $ac('lung') = 4$ and $ac('tonsil') = 2$ as well as its own local costs $lc('organ') = 0$.

In order to determine (un)stable regions in the new version, we need to transfer aggregated costs from O_{old} into O_{new}. We therefore sum up aggregated costs

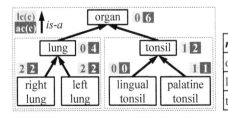

Region Measures

region	abs_size	abs_costs	avg_costs
organ	7	6	0.86
lung	3	4	1.33
tonsil	3	2	0.67

Fig. 1. Example anatomy ontology with regions and local ($lc(c)$) and aggregated ($ac(c)$) concept costs (left). Region measures for example ontology (right).

which belong to the same concept in the old/new version. The new ontology version with aggregated costs is used for further processing. The two version method is generalized for multiple released versions $O_1, \ldots, O_n$ by executing it $n - 1$ times so that we successively determine aggregated costs (for each version change $O_{i-1} \mapsto O_i$) and transfer them to the newest version O_n. In O_n we can apply different measures to detect ontology regions and their change intensities. For further details about the underlying algorithms we refer to [4].

An ontology region OR consists of an ontology concept (region root rc) and its *is-a* subgraph, i.e. it covers all leaf and inner concept changes within this region. For our example in Fig. 1 we can consider the regions 'lung' and 'tonsil' each consisting of three concepts. Note that the complete ontology can also be regarded as a region defined by the ontology root 'organ'. So far, REX provides a set of measures to describe the change intensity of ontology regions. For each OR one can determine its absolute size ($abs\_size(OR)$) w.r.t. the number of concepts. Absolute change costs of an OR ($abs\_costs(OR)$) are represented by the aggregated costs of its root $ac(rc)$. The average change costs per concept in OR can be computed as the fraction of absolute change costs and the region size: $avg\_costs(OR) = \frac{abs\_costs(OR)}{abs\_size(OR)}$. Applying these measures to our example results in the values displayed in Fig. 1 (right). The 'lung' region changed more intensively ($avg\_costs('lung') \approx 1.33$) compared to 'tonsil' ($avg\_costs('tonsil') \approx 0.67$). The overall change intensity of the ontology is $\frac{6}{7} \approx 0.86$.

Trend Discovery for Regions. Using the region discovery method one can determine the most (un)stable regions for a specific time interval. To better monitor region changes over long periods of time and to figure out trends in their evolution, we propose a further method for trend discovery based on sliding windows. The overall procedure **trendDiscovery** looks as follows:

Algorithm 1. trendDiscovery

Input: time interval (t_{start}, t_{end}), ontology O, ontology region of interest
        $OR \in O$, change costs σ, window size ω, step width Δ
Output: time-based stability values $measuredCosts$

1 $t \leftarrow t_{start}$; $measuredCosts \leftarrow \emptyset$;
2 **while** $t + \omega < t_{end}$ **do**
3 | $versions \leftarrow$ getReleasedVersions$(O, (t - \omega, t))$;
4 | $latestVersion \leftarrow$ discoverRegions$(versions, \sigma)$;
5 | $regionCosts \leftarrow$ getStabilityValuesForRegion$(OR, latestVersion)$;
6 | $measuredCosts$.put$((t, regionCosts))$;
7 └ $t \leftarrow t + \Delta$;

8 **return** $measuredCosts$;

The algorithm works on an ontology O, a time interval (t_{start}, t_{end}) and an ontology region of interest OR to be monitored. We further use a sliding window of size ω, a step width Δ and change costs σ. In particular, we successively shift the window beginning at $t_{start} - \omega$ over the time interval until we reach its end t_{end}. In each step we first determine the released ontology versions within the

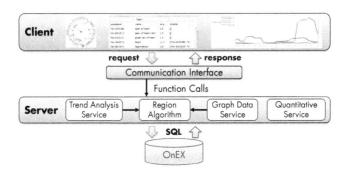

Fig. 2. Three-layered architecture of REX

window (line 3). We then calculate and save the costs (e.g., *avg_costs*) for OR by calling the region discovery algorithm (`discoverRegions`) for the versions within ω. We thus generate a time-based map (line 6) containing information about the change intensity of OR at specific points in time in the defined window. The results are visualized for end users in the *Trend Analysis* component of REX.

3   Infrastructure and Application

REX is based on a three-layered architecture displayed in Fig. 2. The back-end consists of the OnEX repository [6] which currently provides access to up to 1,000 versions of 16 popular life science ontologies. Note that it supports the import of ontologies in different formats such as OWL and OBO. Users can analyze integrated versions with the offered facilities of REX. The server layer is implemented in Java and realizes different services to access ontology versions in OnEX. Moreover, it provides services to calculate the region measures and to perform trend and quantitative analyses. Every service is encapsulated in its own module, such that it is possible to change the region discovery algorithm independently of the other modules. Results are transformed such that the application can visualize ontologies and changing regions in graphs. Based on the existing services we can create further interfaces like web services for programmatic access. The front-end is a platform-independent web application based on the Google Web Toolkit (GWT)[1] and the graph library InfoVis[2]. In the following we discuss the analysis facilities of REX, namely the *Structural Analysis*, *Trend Analysis* and *Quantitative Change Analysis* in more detail.

Structural Analysis. The structural analysis component represents the evolution of regions in an ontology for a specified time interval as a graph (Fig. 3). The component is divided into a *Browser View* as well as a table to search and filter results (*Table View*). First the user needs to specify the ontology name

---

[1] Google Web Toolkit: `http://developers.google.com/web-toolkit/`
[2] InfoVis Toolkit: `http://philogb.github.io/jit/`

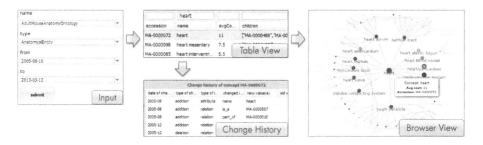

Fig. 3. Structural Analysis component

and the time period to review in the *Input* form. The system then performs the region discovery algorithms and generates a graph to visualize the results (*Browser View*). Each node in the graph represents an ontology concept, *is-a* relationships are displayed as edges between the nodes. The layout is circular and displays a concept and its near neighborhood, i.e. its descendants and parent nodes (either with or without labels). Users can easily identify interesting sub regions by selecting a concept in the graph (*Browser View*) or in the *Table View*. This concept is then shown as the central node in the *Browser View*. It is possible to navigate in both directions through the ontology. For instance, if one is interested in a specific sub region and its content, one clicks on the node and the graph will display the sub region in more detail. In contrast, one can also navigate to a more general concept (surrounded by blue circles) to see sibling regions of the current one. The colors signal the measured change intensity (*avg_costs*) of a region. Red stays for high change intensity whereby green is used to mark stable regions. Thus, users can easily figure out where (un)stable regions are located. We provide two coloring schemes: (1) interval-based grouping or (2) equal distribution between min/max *avg_costs*. When clicking on a specific concept in the graph one can get further information like the accession number, concept name/label or the measured *avg_costs* in a pop up window.

In general the number of concepts and relationships in an ontology is very high. Thus, it is difficult to recognize interesting regions only by browsing through the graph especially for large ontologies. Moreover, users may be interested in the change intensity of specific regions. The *Table View* therefore allows users to filter and sort ontology regions by their accession number, name and *avg_costs*. In particular, search criteria can be specified in the head of the table to find regions of interest. For instance, one can filter out all regions in the Adult Mouse Anatomy Ontology containing the name 'heart'. Users can simply select their region of interest in the table and move to the *Browser View* for its visualization. To get a more detailed view of occurred changes, users can request the local *Change History* of a selected concept at the bottom of the table.

Quantitative Change Analysis. To get information about how many changes occurred in an ontology for a specific time interval REX offers the quantitative change analysis component (Fig. 4 left). Users can generate diagrams to see the differences between released ontology versions in statistical (quantitative)

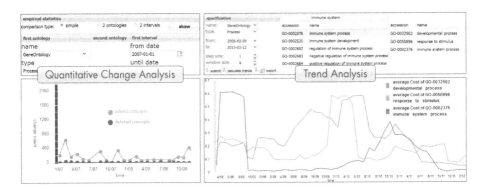

Fig. 4. Trend and Quantitative Change Analysis components

form, i.e., we count and visualize how many changes ($addC$, $delC$, $addR$, $delR$) occurred. In particular, users can display the number of changes in one ontology for a specific time interval, e.g., GO Biological Processes in 2011. Moreover, one can compare the evolution of two different ontologies for a specified time interval or compare two different time intervals for the same ontology. Users can thus identify interesting ontologies and time periods for later region analyses.

Trend Analysis. The trend analysis component can be used to study and compare the long-term evolution of selected regions (Fig. 4 right). Users first need to specify the ontology, the time interval (first and last version) and the window size and step width (number of versions). Next they are able to select regions of their interest either by searching the respective accession number / concept name or by choosing from top-level concepts of the ontology. REX executes the proposed `trendDiscovery` algorithm to measure the avg_costs for the selected regions at different points in time. The results are converted into a line chart which displays the trend of the measured avg_costs for each region over time. Users are thus able to compare the change intensity for different regions of interest within one diagram. Of course, the interpretation of trend results is up to the user and depends on the application scenario. Some regions may be of high research interest and are thus continuously adapted (constantly high avg_costs). Other regions have been adapted heavily in the past and become stable after a while. By contrast, some long-term stable regions might have just been of low interest in the past and need future development.

4   Conclusion and Future Work

REX provides interactive access to information about the evolution of life science ontologies. Users can explore (un)stable ontology regions by different workflows. The knowledge about changing ontology regions can be used to support ontology-based algorithms and analysis. Furthermore, the development of large life science ontologies can be monitored with REX, i.e., developers and project coordinators can inform themselves about ongoing work in different ontology parts. For future, work we plan to extend REX such that users are able to perform region analysis on their individual ontologies and can apply different cost models. We further like to build a web service interface such that algorithms can directly access the region analysis algorithms.

Acknowledgment. This work is funded by the European Social Fund and the Free State of Saxony (E-Science Network Sachsen).

References

1. Bodenreider, O., Stevens, R.: Bio-ontologies: current trends and future directions. Briefings in Bioinformatics 7(3) (2006)
2. Groß, A., Hartung, M., Prüfer, K., et al.: Impact of ontology evolution on functional analyses. Bioinformatics 28(20) (2012)
3. Groza, T., Tudorache, T., Dumontier, M.: Commentary: State of the art and open challenges in community-driven knowledge curation. Journal of Biomedical Informatics 46(1) (2013)
4. Hartung, M., Gross, A., Kirsten, T., Rahm, E.: Discovering Evolving Regions in Life Science Ontologies. In: Lambrix, P., Kemp, G. (eds.) DILS 2010. LNCS, vol. 6254, pp. 19–34. Springer, Heidelberg (2010)
5. Hartung, M., Gross, A., Rahm, E.: CODEX: exploration of semantic changes between ontology versions. Bioinformatics 28(6) (2012)
6. Hartung, M., Kirsten, T., Gross, A., Rahm, E.: OnEX: Exploring changes in life science ontologies. BMC Bioinformatics 10(1) (2009)
7. Hartung, M., Terwilliger, J.F., Rahm, E.: Recent Advances in Schema and Ontology Evolution. In: Schema Matching and Mapping. Springer, Heidelberg (2011)
8. Lambrix, P., Tan, H., Jakoniene, V., Strömbäck, L.: Biological ontologies. In: Semantic Web. Springer, Heidelberg (2007)
9. Malone, J., Stevens, R.: Measuring the level of activity in community built bio-ontologies. Journal of Biomedical Informatics 46(1) (2013)
10. Noy, N.F., Shah, N.H., Whetzel, P., et al.: BioPortal: ontologies and integrated data resources at the click of a mouse. Nucleic Acids Research 37(suppl. 2) (2009)
11. Park, J.C., Kim, T., Park, J.: Monitoring the evolutionary aspect of the gene ontology to enhance predictability and usability. BMC Bioinformatics 9 (2008)
12. Park, Y.R., Park, C.H., Kim, J.H.: GOChase: correcting errors from Gene Ontology-based annotations for gene products. Bioinformatics 21(6) (2005)
13. Sioutos, N., De Coronado, S., Haber, M.W., et al.: NCI Thesaurus: a semantic model integrating cancer-related clinical and molecular information. Journal of Biomedical Informatics 40(1) (2007)
14. Smith, B., Ashburner, M., Rosse, C., et al.: The OBO Foundry: coordinated evolution of ontologies to support biomedical data integration. Nature Biotechnology 25(11) (2007)
15. Subramanian, A., Tamayo, P., Mootha, V.K., et al.: Gene set enrichment analysis: a knowledge-based approach for interpreting genome-wide expression profiles. PNAS 102(43) (2005)
16. Tudorache, T., Noy, N.F., Tu, S., Musen, M.A.: Supporting collaborative ontology development in protégé. In: Sheth, A.P., Staab, S., Dean, M., Paolucci, M., Maynard, D., Finin, T., Thirunarayan, K. (eds.) ISWC 2008. LNCS, vol. 5318, pp. 17–32. Springer, Heidelberg (2008)

Towards Visualizing the Alignment of Large Biomedical Ontologies

Catia Pesquita[1], Daniel Faria[1], Emanuel Santos[1],
Jean-Marc Neefs[2], and Francisco M. Couto[1]

[1] Dept. de Informática, Faculdade de Ciências, Universidade de Lisboa, Portugal
[2] Janssen Pharmaceutical Companies of Johnson & Johnson
`cpesquita@di.fc.ul.pt`

Abstract. To successfully integrate biomedical data it is crucial to establish meaningful relationships between the ontologies used to annotate this data. Recent developments in ontology alignment techniques, including our AgreementMakerLight system, have been successful in matching very large biomedical ontologies. However the visualization of these alignments is still a challenge.

We have developed a graphical user interface for AgreementMakerLight that follows its core focus on computational efficiency and the handling of very large ontologies. It allows non-expert users to easily align biomedical ontologies, offering a wide selection of matching strategies and algorithms, with a particular focus on the use of external background knowledge. The visualization of the resulting alignment is based on linked subgraphs which are generated according to search queries over the full graph composed by the matched ontologies and the mappings between them. This strategy decreases the need for computational resources and improves the visualization experience, by letting the user focus on selected areas of the alignment.

Keywords: Ontology Matching, Ontology Alignment, Alignment Visualization, Large Ontologies, Biomedical Ontologies.

1 Introduction

Biomedical ontologies and controlled vocabularies are now a widely used technology to support the annotation of life sciences datasets. However, only by establishing meaningful connections across the concepts from various ontologies can we fully explore the knowledge they contain. Ontology matching techniques can accomplish this since they create mappings (i.e., correspondences) between semantically related entities belonging to different ontologies [1]. Ontology matching systems usually employ several ontology matching techniques both at the element and structural level which are then combined to produce a final alignment.

There are several challenges in matching biomedical ontologies, which arise from their characteristics. For instance, one of the main components of biomedical ontologies is their textual information, in the form of labels, synonyms and

H. Galhardas and E. Rahm (Eds.): DILS 2014, LNBI 8574, pp. 104–111, 2014.

definitions. Successful ontology matching systems need to be able to handle this richness, and also the inherent complexity of biomedical terminology. Furthermore, the domains covered by biomedical ontologies are frequently very large and detailed, with many biomedical ontologies possessing tens of thousands of classes dedicated to highly specific areas such as genomics, phenotypes or cellular structures. However, there are also opportunities within the biomedical domain such as the abundance of scientific literature or the availability of many related biomedical ontologies. Although there is a community effort to ensure orthogonality between ontologies as much as possible [2], there is still a significant overlap between many of them. In a recent visualization effort of the mappings between BioPortal [3] ontologies it has been shown that there are 254 ontologies with at least one mapping to another ontology. These mappings have been created through strict string matching and thus represent only a fraction of the true overlap between ontologies. In fact, at the time of writing this paper there were 373 ontologies in BioPortal and about 13 million mappings.

In order to address these issues, recent ontology matching systems have begun to include more elaborate strategies, such as creating highly efficient data structures or modularization approaches to handle very large ontologies [4,5], tailoring of string similarity metrics [6] and exploration of different synonym types [7], ontology repair techniques to ensure the coherence of the alignments [5,4], and the use of external resources and ontologies to increase the amount of available knowledge to support matching [5,8].

An important feature of ontology matching systems is the ability to visualize the alignments between the ontologies, particularly in the biomedical domain where many of the end-users are not computer science experts. There are two main purposes in alignment visualization: supporting the navigation and inspection of mappings; and supporting interactive matching, whereby users can mark mappings as correct or incorrect, and even add new mappings [9,4,10]. These tasks are usually supported by two visual paradigms: trees and graphs [11]. Trees are particularly intuitive representations of hierarchical relations, however they are unable to represent multiple inheritance, and have to resort to duplication of classes, distorting the model. Graphs can handle both multiple inheritance and non-hierarchical relations, but can be less intuitive to use, particularly if the number of nodes shown is high. A recent evaluation of tree vs. graph based visualization has investigated the impact of individual ontology representation on the task of manual mapping evaluation [12]. In this study ontologies were represented either as trees or graphs and testers were given a list of mappings to evaluate. The results showed that trees are better suited to support list-checking activities, such as the evaluation of mappings, but graphs are more suitable to provide an overview, and thus better at supporting the creation of new mappings. Furthermore, for very large ontologies, with great depth and a large number of descendants per node, users struggle to preserve a mental model of the hierarchy when using trees, since the number of expandable nodes can be overwhelming. Graphs can partially circumvent this by allowing users to pan to areas of interest, however visualization of a large number of nodes is also an issue.

However, ontology alignment visualization systems should consider not only how to represent the ontologies, but also the mappings between them. Furthermore, there are additional challenges posed by biomedical ontologies: (1) biomedical ontologies are typically large, sometimes with tens of thousands of classes; (2) many biomedical ontologies can have multiple inheritance or possess more than one kind of hierarchical relation (e.g., a taxonomy as well as a partonomy); and (3) non-hierarchical relations are also common, e.g. *regulates*, *has_substrate*, *has_role*, *participates_in*, etc. However, the matching of very large ontologies has only recently begun to be addressed by systems, and as a result current ontology matching systems with visualization capabilities are not well suited to either match or visualize very large ontologies with these characteristics.

In previous work we have developed a novel ontology matching system, AgreementMakerLight [5], derived from AgreementMaker, but specifically tailored to match very large ontologies. Here we present a graphical user interface for AgreementMakerLight, which supports the matching of large ontologies with several distinct parameters, including the use of background knowledge. The GUI also supports a graph-based visualization of mappings, that highlights the integration of both ontologies in a modular fashion.

2   Related Work

Most ontology alignment visualization systems display ontologies as trees, which the user can navigate, while mappings are shown as lines between the two ontologies [13,14] or displayed in a table [15]. We have surveyed three freely and currently available ontology matching systems with visualization capabilities: AgreementMaker, COMA 3.0 and Optima.

AgreementMaker [13] represents ontologies as indented trees on side by side scroll-enabled panes. A mapping between two classes is represented by a straight line indicating the similarity score of the mapping. There is support for the visualization of several alignments over the same ontologies, using different colored lines for mappings of different alignments. When clicking on a node, users can see the properties of the corresponding class in a separate pane. However, AgreementMaker is unable to handle ontologies with tens of thousands of classes.

COMA 3.0 Community Edition [14] depicts ontologies as indented graphs in side-by-side scroll-enabled panels. When a node is clicked, the main label is shown along with the path to the root node in the form of coma separated labels. Mappings are colored according to their score. It is possible to compute different matching workflows over the same input ontologies, but you can only visualize one at a time. Different matching results can be merged or intersected, and their differences can be also be calculated. Furthermore, the tool is not optimized to handle large ontologies. Neither COMA 3.0 nor AgreementMaker allow for the visualization of non-hierarchical relations, nor of multiple inheritance.

Optima [16] displays each ontology as a graph in a window without zoom capabilities, which severely limits its usability for large ontologies, since all nodes need to fit in a constrained area. Mapped nodes are highlighted, and when clicked, their label is shown and when double-clicked the matched node label in the other ontology appears. There is no graphical representation of mappings, nor any listing. Furthermore, the matching technique employed by Optima is also unsuitable to handle large ontologies.

3   AgreementMakerLight

3.1   Framework

The AgreementMakerLight (AML) is a lightweight framework for ontology matching based on the AgreementMaker system, which has been optimized to handle the matching of larger ontologies. Like AgreementMaker, the AML ontology matching module was designed with flexibility and extensibility in mind, and thus allows for the inclusion of virtually any matching algorithm. A key component of AML is the use of background knowledge sources which have been shown to improve the alignment of biomedical ontologies, as evidenced by AML achieving top results in several OAEI 2013 tracks [17].

3.2   Graphical User Interface

The graphical user interface of AML is divided in two areas: a Resource Panel where information about the ontologies and the alignment is shown (e.g.: number of classes, properties, mappings and performance metrics against a reference alignment), and a Mapping Viewer dedicated to the graph visualization of ontologies and mappings (Figure 1).

AML-GUI allows the user to load ontologies in OWL or RDFS and then opt between loading a precomputed alignment (encoded in RDF or as a simple tab-separated text file) and matching the ontologies. There are three pre-defined matchers to choose from: a simple Lexical Matcher, the AML matcher and the OAEI 2013 matcher. The Lexical Matcher is based on name and synonym string identity and is very efficient and generally precise. The AML matcher is an ensemble of string and lexical matching algorithms, with the option to choose several background knowledge sources to use in the matching process (see Figure 2). The OAEI 2013 matcher corresponds to the AML configuration used in OAEI 2013. All matchers have the option to set a cardinality for the alignment (strict one-to-one, permissive one-to-one and many-to-many), and also a threshold to select mappings to include in the final alignment. Both of the latter matchers have the option to perform a repair of the final alignment [18]. Finally, the user can also evaluate the produced alignment against a reference standard, and save it either in RDF or as a tab-separated text file. Once an alignment has been loaded or computed, the user can access a mapping in three different ways: by iterating over all mappings, via the next/previous mapping option; by selecting a mapping from the list of all mappings; or by querying the alignment for a search term contained in the name of a participant ontology class. This search is supported by an auto-complete function.

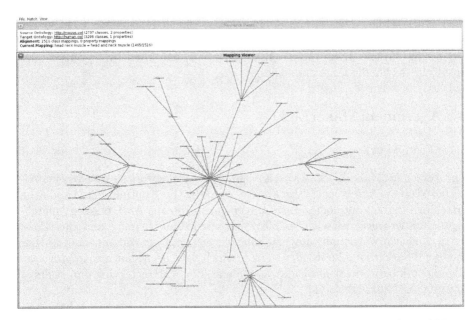

Fig. 1. Visualization of a mapping between anatomical ontologies in AML-GUI

4 Visualizing Ontology Alignments

AML uses a graph to represent the mapped classes and their neighborhood, which is implemented using the Gephi API [19]. Once the user has selected a mapping to visualize, she can further specify the characteristics of its graph representation, by indicating whether the graph should show ancestor and descendant classes, and the distance between the classes involved in the selected mapping and their ancestors/descendants (from one to a maximum of five edges of distance). By default, AML shows both ancestors and descendants at a distance of two. Both ontologies are represented in the same graph, nodes and edges of the source ontology in red and of the target ontology in blue. Nodes are labeled with the classes main labels or names. Ontology edges are labeled with their relation type, except in the case of subsumption relations, which have no label. Directed edges are represented as arrows. Mappings are represented as yellow edges and labeled with their confidence score. Equivalence mappings are represented as double-edged arrows. All mappings between the ontology classes in the selected neighborhood are shown. The user can pan and zoom the graph, and at any time change the visualization options for the selected mapping, generating a new graph.

The following example focuses on the mapping between two classes of the Mouse and Human anatomy ontologies used in OAEI: "head/neck muscle" and "Head and Neck Muscle". Figure 3 shows the representation of the mapping in AgreementMaker. Mapped classes are shown as colored nodes, and the mapping as a line between nodes. It is possible to see the direct descendants and ancestors of one of the mapped classes, which are also colored when they are mapped.

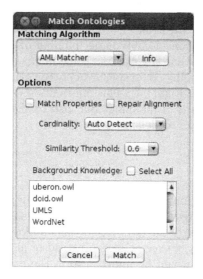

Fig. 2. Configuration window for the AML matcher

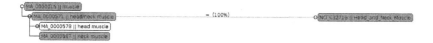

Fig. 3. Visualization of a mapping between anatomical ontologies in AgreementMaker

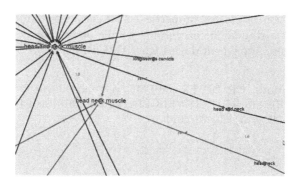

Fig. 4. Detail of a mapping between partonomy classes in anatomical ontologies in AML-GUI

However, it is not possible to see the neighborhood classes for both ontologies at the same time, and likewise it is not possible to see the mappings in this area.

Figure 1 shows the same mapping in AML, with default settings. In the shown ontology subgraphs, there are four other mappings, both between ancestors and descendants of the selected classes. The graph representation allows the observation of several characteristics of the neighboring region of the mapping which are not apparent in the AgreementMaker visualization: the Human Anatomy ontology (in blue) contains a considerably larger number of classes in the neighborhood, half of the Mouse Anatomy classes can be mapped to a Human Anatomy class, and one of the mappings is established between classes that are part of the partonomy hierarchy (see Figure 4). This information can be valuable not only to evaluate the correctness of mappings but also to shed light on how regions around mapped classes are modelled.

5   Conclusions

Visualizing ontology alignments is a key feature to support user validation. In AML we focused on addressing the challenges in visualizing biomedical ontologies alignments, particularly the large size of the ontologies and the existence of several types of relations between classes. Instead of allowing the visualization of full ontologies, which would be impractical in the case of very large ontologies, we have chosen to focus our visualization on the mappings. By selecting a particular mapping, users are shown a single graph composed of modules of both ontologies connected through their mappings. With this approach, we hope to better support the understanding of related areas within aligned ontologies, contrasting with the currently common approach of using linked trees in separate panes. Furthermore, by being graph-based, AML allows the visualization of several types of relations between ontology classes, including the cases of multiple-inheritance, which can be crucial to evaluate the validity of mappings.

As future work, we plan to include dynamic graphs, graph color customization, and inspection of classes properties. AML is open-source and currently available both as a standalone executable jar file and as an Eclipse project at https://github.com/AgreementMakerLight/AML-Project.

Acknowledgements. CP, DF, ES and FMC were funded by the Portuguese FCT through the SOMER project (PTDC/EIA-EIA/119119/2010) and LaSIGE Strategic Project, ref. PEst-OE/EEI/UI0408/2014.

References

1. Euzenat, J., Shvaiko, P.: Ontology matching, vol. 18. Springer, Berlin (2007)
2. Smith, B., Ashburner, M., Rosse, C., Bard, J., Bug, W., Ceusters, W., Goldberg, L., Eilbeck, K., Ireland, A., Mungall, C., et al.: The OBO Foundry: coordinated evolution of ontologies to support biomedical data integration. Nature Biotechnology 25(11), 1251–1255 (2007)
3. Kocbek, S., Perret, J.L., Kim, J.D.: Visual presentation of mappings between biomedical ontologies. In: SWAT4LS (2012)
4. Jiménez-Ruiz, E., Grau, B.C., Zhou, Y., Horrocks, I.: Large-scale interactive ontology matching: Algorithms and implementation. In: ECAI, vol. 242, pp. 444–449 (2012)

5. Faria, D., Pesquita, C., Santos, E., Palmonari, M., Cruz, I.F., Couto, F.M.: The agreementMakerLight ontology matching system. In: Meersman, R., Panetto, H., Dillon, T., Eder, J., Bellahsene, Z., Ritter, N., De Leenheer, P., Dou, D. (eds.) ODBASE 2013. LNCS, vol. 8185, pp. 527–541. Springer, Heidelberg (2013)
6. Cheatham, M., Hitzler, P.: String similarity metrics for ontology alignment. In: Alani, H., Kagal, L., Fokoue, A., Groth, P., Biemann, C., Parreira, J.X., Aroyo, L., Noy, N., Welty, C., Janowicz, K. (eds.) ISWC 2013, Part II. LNCS, vol. 8219, pp. 294–309. Springer, Heidelberg (2013)
7. Pesquita, C., Faria, D., Stroe, C., Santos, E., Cruz, I.F., Couto, F.M.: What's in a 'nym'? Synonyms in Biomedical Ontology Matching. In: Alani, H., Kagal, L., Fokoue, A., Groth, P., Biemann, C., Parreira, J.X., Aroyo, L., Noy, N., Welty, C., Janowicz, K. (eds.) ISWC 2013, Part I. LNCS, vol. 8218, pp. 526–541. Springer, Heidelberg (2013)
8. Hartung, M., Gross, A., Kirsten, T., Rahm, E.: Effective mapping composition for biomedical ontologies. In: Semantic Interoperability in Medical Informatics (SIMI-2012), Workshop at ESWC, vol. 12 (2012)
9. Paulheim, H., Hertling, S., Ritze, D.: Towards evaluating interactive ontology matching tools. In: Cimiano, P., Corcho, O., Presutti, V., Hollink, L., Rudolph, S. (eds.) ESWC 2013. LNCS, vol. 7882, pp. 31–45. Springer, Heidelberg (2013)
10. Cruz, I.F., Stroe, C., Palmonari, M.: Interactive user feedback in ontology matching using signature vectors. In: 2012 IEEE 28th International Conference on Data Engineering (ICDE), pp. 1321–1324. IEEE (2012)
11. Granitzer, M., Sabol, V., Onn, K.W., Lukose, D., Tochtermann, K.: Ontology alignmenta survey with focus on visually supported semi-automatic techniques. Future Internet 2(3), 238–258 (2010)
12. Fu, B., Noy, N.F., Storey, M.-A.: Indented tree or graph? A usability study of ontology visualization techniques in the context of class mapping evaluation. In: Alani, H., Kagal, L., Fokoue, A., Groth, P., Biemann, C., Parreira, J.X., Aroyo, L., Noy, N., Welty, C., Janowicz, K. (eds.) ISWC 2013, Part I. LNCS, vol. 8218, pp. 117–134. Springer, Heidelberg (2013)
13. Cruz, I.F., Sunna, W.: Structural Alignment Methods with Applications to Geospatial Ontologies. Transactions in GIS, Special Issue on Semantic Similarity Measurement and Geospatial Applications 12(6), 683–711 (2008)
14. Massmann, S., Raunich, S., Aumüller, D., Arnold, P., Rahm, E.: Evolution of the COMA match system. Ontology Matching 49 (2011)
15. Ngo, D., Bellahsene, Z.: YAM++: A multi-strategy based approach for ontology matching task. In: ten Teije, A., Völker, J., Handschuh, S., Stuckenschmidt, H., d'Acquin, M., Nikolov, A., Aussenac-Gilles, N., Hernandez, N. (eds.) EKAW 2012. LNCS, vol. 7603, pp. 421–425. Springer, Heidelberg (2012)
16. Thayasivam, U., Doshi, P.: Optima results for oaei 2011. In: Proc. of 6th OM Workshop, pp. 204–211 (2011)
17. Grau, B.C., Dragisic, Z., Eckert, K., Euzenat, J., Ferrara, A., Granada, R., Ivanova, V., Jiménez-Ruiz, E., Kempf, A.O., Lambrix, P., et al.: Results of the ontology alignment evaluation initiative 2013. In: Proc. 8th ISWC workshop on ontology matching (OM), pp. 61–100 (2013)
18. Santos, E., Faria, D., Pesquita, C., Couto, F.: Ontology alignment repair through modularization and confidence-based heuristics. arXiv preprint arXiv:1307.5322 (2013)
19. Bastian, M., Heymann, S., Jacomy, M.: Gephi: an open source software for exploring and manipulating networks. In: ICWSM, pp. 361–362 (2009)

Discovering Relations between Indirectly Connected Biomedical Concepts

Dirk Weissenborn, Michael Schroeder, and George Tsatsaronis

Biotechnology Center, Technische Universität Dresden, Dresden, Germany
{dirk.weissenborn,ms,george.tsatsaronis}@biotec.tu-dresden.de

Abstract. The complexity and scale of the knowledge in the biomedical domain has motivated research work towards mining heterogeneous data from structured and unstructured knowledge bases. Towards this direction, it is necessary to combine facts in order to formulate hypotheses or draw conclusions about the domain concepts. In this work we attempt to address this problem by using indirect knowledge connecting two concepts in a graph to identify hidden relations between them. The graph represents concepts as vertices and relations as edges, stemming from structured (ontologies) and unstructured (text) data. In this graph we attempt to mine path patterns which potentially characterize a biomedical relation. For our experimental evaluation we focus on two frequent relations, namely *"has target"*, and *"may treat"*. Our results suggest that relation discovery using indirect knowledge is possible, with an AUC that can reach up to 0.8. Finally, analysis of the results indicates that the models can successfully learn expressive path patterns for the examined relations.

Keywords: Relation Discovery, Biomedical Concepts, Text Mining.

1 Introduction

Knowledge discovery in the biomedical domain has been a subject of study for many years; yet, the increasing complexity of the task due to the size and number of biomedical resources has been motivating the work in the area towards efficient, scalable and interpretable, in terms of results, methodologies. Two examples of how fast the biomedical resources grow are illustrated in Figure 1.

Besides the obstacles that the scale of the data brings into the task of extracting information, combining knowledge together to cover as many aspects as possible is also an issue. For example, typical information extraction techniques focusing on drugs aim at extracting targets, adverse effects and indications, which cannot be achieved by limiting the applied methods to a small fragment of drug related information. Hence, it is necessary to combine facts in order to formulate hypotheses or draw conclusions about the domain concepts.

In this work we address this problem by using indirect knowledge connecting two concepts to discover hidden relations between them. To find such indirect connections, we represent knowledge via a graph comprising concepts as vertices

H. Galhardas and E. Rahm (Eds.): DILS 2014, LNBI 8574, pp. 112–119, 2014.
© Springer International Publishing Switzerland 2014

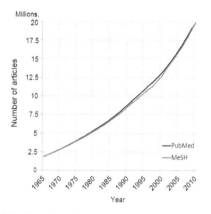
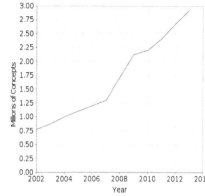

(a) Growth of PubMed indexed scientific literature since 1965

(b) Growth of the UMLS Metathesaurus in the past decade

Fig. 1. Growth over time of two biomedical resources

and labeled edges connecting the concepts. Edges are created by either extracting explicit knowledge from structured databases, or by analyzing unstructured textual data. This provides a simple framework that is easy to interpret and constitutes the integration of heterogeneous data easy. In order to perform relation discovery on top of this representation, we are using supervised machine learning to learn path patterns that characterize these relations. For the evaluation of our approach we study the ability of this modeling to discover *has target* relations between drugs and proteins/genes, and *may treat* relations drugs and diseases. The results demonstrate the feasibility of the task using the suggested approach, which manages to extract characteristic patterns for these relations.

2   Relation Discovery between Indirectly Connected Biomedical Concepts

Most work on knowledge discovery in natural language text focuses on extracting relations between two concepts mentioned in one sentence. This is very important for many applications such as the curation of databases. However, Swanson [1] has shown the potential of combining facts from different sources to discover new, yet unknown knowledge.

Recently, many studies [2,3] have been conducted on discovering hidden relations between concepts based on statistical analysis. This approach differs from ours in that linguistic information is not exploited. Another approach was taken with BioLiterate [4] using probabilistic inference, which may discover relations between concepts that do not necessarily co-occur in the same abstracts. In contrast to this work, their approach is based on a collection of manually constructed rules that map linguistic constructs onto a probabilistic reasoning system. Furthermore, the metathesaurus and the semantic network of the UMLS resource have been used extensively in the past to identify relationships between concepts, e.g., in [5] for the purposes of auditing associative relations. However, most of these works rely in that the semantics of the associative relations should be defined explicitly in order to be extracted, in contrast to our work which does not depend on such definitions. Arguably the most similar work to ours is the work of Lao et al. [6], as the goal and approach of their study is similar. An open domain, web-scale corpus is used to train a classifier with a huge amount of training examples represented in a very large feature space. However, the requirements of our work, namely a limited amount of training data and a much smaller textual corpus, require a different way of modeling and training.

2.1   Knowledge Sources and Representation

In this work we are using the Metathesaurus from the *Unified Medical Language System* (UMLS) and DrugBank as our structured knowledge bases, and MEDLINE as our unstructured knowledge resource. For the inclusion of the latter in our work, we are using an already annotated version of the MEDLINE documents with the MetaMap program [7].

Both structured and unstructured knowledge is represented by a directed, edge-labeled graph $G = (C, R)$, consisting of a set of concepts as vertices C and a set of labeled edges R. We define $(c_i, c_j) \in R_l \Leftrightarrow (c_i, l, c_j) \in R$, where $R_l \subseteq C \times C$ is an l-labeled binary relation. We allow a triple to occur more than once in R, which means that R is actually a multiset. A path P in G of length n is an n-tuple of vertices $P = (c_1, ..., c_n)$, where $\forall i, 1 \leq i < n : \exists l \in L : (c_i, l, c_{i+1}) \in R$, meaning that there must be at least one edge between the concepts c_i and c_{i+1} for every i.

Representing the structured knowledge sources, such as UMLS and DrugBank, in such a graph is straightforward; these sources already contain labeled relations $R_l \subseteq C \times C$. The information of all those R_l, i.e., their concept pairs (c_i, c_j) together with their label l, can directly be inserted into the graph by adding each c_i and c_j to C and all corresponding triples (c_i, l, c_j) as edges to R.

In contrast to the structured knowledge representation, extracting such triples from unstructured textual data is more difficult, because it entails a series of pre-processing steps, such as annotation of the text with biomedical concepts, and meta-analysis and filtering of the annotations. However, since we are using the already annotated version of MEDLINE with UMLS concepts, this task is reduced to extracting only the relations between concepts found in one sentence. In that respect, previous work on relation extraction, e.g., [8], has shown that the *dependency path* between two concepts in a sentence typically contains all necessary information to recognize a specific underlying relation between them. A dependency path is a path in a *dependency tree*, which is a syntactic construct of a sentence. Each node of a dependency tree represents a token (word or symbol) of the underlying sentence and each arch represents a dependency between two tokens of the sentence. Hence, we extract triples from sentences when we find a pair of concepts connected by a dependency path that contains at least one verb form. If the dependency path does not contain any verb form, we assume that there is no relation present in this sentence. If we find more than one verb form on the dependency path which are part of two distinct sub-sentences connected by a conjunction, we assume that there is no direct relation between such concept pairs present and discard them as well. Sequences of conjunctions and appositions are removed from the dependency paths. If there is a negated noun or verb form present on the dependency path, the whole path will be treated as negated as well. Once a pair of concepts (c_i, c_j) is extracted from a sentence together with its (cleaned) dependency path d_k, a triple (c_i, d_k, c_j) can be inserted into the knowledge graph G the same way as for structured knowledge.

2.2   Methodology

Graph Path Discovery: To extract paths for a concept pair (c_s, c_t) to a maximum path length m, a bidirectional search is performed. Searching is, thus, done by starting from both vertices c_s and c_t until a maximum path length of $\lfloor \frac{m+1}{2} \rfloor$ from each side is reached. During the search, paths are explored stochastically in a random walk, but in most cases the number of neighbors is not very high and, hence, every neighbor will be explored.

Modeling: Encoding a graph path $P = (c_1, ..., c_n)$ requires an encoding of each connection (c_i, c_{i+1}) in P as a feature vector $f_{(c_i, c_{i+1})}$, resulting in a sequence of feature vectors of length $n - 1$. The feature vector $f_{(c_i, c_{i+1})}$ is defined as the sum of all feature vectors of each relation label l occurring between c_i and c_{i+1}.

The simplest way of encoding a relation label l is the one-of-N encoding, where only the l-dimension of the feature vector has value 1 and all others have 0. This encoding, however, is very poor because it does not take into account semantic similarities and synonymy information between the relation labels. This in turn leads to an explosion of the feature space. We address this problem by encoding the relations in a much smaller semantic feature space. For this purpose, there are several techniques that may be applied, e.g., *latent semantic analysis* (LSA), *reflective random indexing* (RRI), *the generalization of principle component analysis* (gPCA) or *latent dirichlet allocation* (LDA, [9]).

The basic idea for constructing a semantic space of relations is to consider a pair of connected vertices, i.e., concepts, (c_i, c_j) in G as a document $d_{i,j}$ and all labels of all edges, i.e., relations, between them as words occurring in $d_{i,j}$. Using this transformation for all connected concept pairs of G, the above mentioned algorithms can be used natively to construct semantic feature vectors of a specified size for each relation label. In our implementation we used *LDA* because its underlying model fits well to the problem. This way, f_l using *LDA* features is defined as the conditional probability distribution over all possible latent topics t given label l, as shown in the following equation.

$$f_l^t = p(t|l)$$
$$p(t|l) \propto p(t) \cdot p(l|t) \tag{1}$$

where f_l^t is the value of the t-th dimension of f_l, and $p(t)$, $p(l|t)$ are taken from the trained *LDA* model.

Given the above, the creation of the feature vector for an indirectly connected pair is done as follows: given a set of graph paths $\mathfrak{P}_{c_s,c_t}$ between the concepts c_s and c_t, the feature vector f_{c_s,c_t} is defined as the sum of the feature vectors f_P representing all paths $P \in \mathfrak{P}_{c_s,c_t}$. The feature vector of a path $P = (c_1, ..., c_n)$ is calculated from its corresponding sequence $f_{(c_i,c_{i+1})} \in \mathbb{R}^N$ of feature vectors by projecting their outer product which is a $(n-1)$-dimensional matrix to a vector representation. This is described by the following equation.

$$f_{c_s,c_t} = \sum_{P \in \mathfrak{P}_{c_s,c_t}} f_P \tag{2}$$

$$f_P = \pi(f_{(c_1,c_2)} \otimes \cdots \otimes f_{(c_{n-1},c_n)}) \tag{3}$$

Training: Let $R_l \subset C \times C$, be a relation of label l. A model for relation label l is trained with a set of positive training examples $E_l^+ \subseteq R_l$ and negative training examples $E_l^- \subset C \times C$. E_l^- is constructed from E_l^+ by pairing all source concepts of E_l^+ with a random target concept of E_l^+, ensuring that $E_l^+ \cap E_l^- = \emptyset$. Training of logistic regression is performed using gradient ascent on the likelihood function by employing *LBFGS* with *L2*-regularization. The *LDA* model is trained using the efficient sparse stochastic inference algorithm [10].

3   Experimental Evaluation

For the purposes of evaluating experimentally the suggested approach, we constructed a graph as explained previously, and created two benchmark datasets for two relations; *has target* and *may treat*. The graph is used to extract paths between pairs of concepts in these relations, which in turn form the basis for the feature vectors generation.

3.1   Experimental Setup

The constructed graph, resulting after pruning of infrequently occurring concepts and relations[1], contains $95,158$ vertices, which are all the UMLS concepts occurring in the textual data, approximately 39 million edges created from the analysis of the unstructured data (MEDLINE documents), and around 2.8 million edges stemming from the structured sources. The average degree is approximately 880 considering both incoming and outgoing direction of edges. In terms of relation labels, the graph contains approximately $104,953$ distinct labels, where each label occurs on average 5 times, connecting around 30 million pairs of vertices.

With regards to the used datasets, the first dataset contains 410 concept pairs of the *may treat* relation taken from the UMLS. It covers a wide range of diseases,

---

[1] Concepts occurring less than 50 times and relations occurring less than 40 times were removed.

Table 1. Examples of highly weighted plain path features for the *has target* (former) and the *may treat* (latter) relations

highly weighted feature	explanation
$(\xrightarrow{dep} induce \xleftarrow{prep} in \xleftarrow{pobj})$, $(\xrightarrow{pobj}$ $in \xrightarrow{prep} express \xleftarrow{nsubjpass})$	The substance is induced into something, in which the target (gene/protein) is expressed.
$(\xrightarrow{pobj} by \xrightarrow{agent} suppress \xleftarrow{nsubjpass})$, $(\xrightarrow{nsubj} increase \xleftarrow{prep} at \xleftarrow{pobj})$	The drug suppresses something that is increased by the disease.

Table 2. Impact of maximum path lengths

dataset	length	AUC		accuracy (precision, recall)	
		plain	*lda*	*plain*	*lda*
may treat	3-3	0.61	0.73	0.63 (0.63, 0.61)	0.69 (0.76, 0.63)
	3-4	0.62	0.75	0.62 (0.67, 0.49)	0.70 (0.71, 0.69)
has target	3-3	0.78	0.72	0.75 (0.87, 0.59)	0.68 (0.74, 0.60)
	3-4	0.80	0.70	0.77 (0.84, 0.66)	0.66 (0.70, 0.58)

and every concept only appears once in the dataset. The second set consists of 740 pairs of the *has target* relation, extracted from DrugBank and mapped to UMLS. Negative examples in both cases are extracted as explained in the previous section. Finally, all models and training algorithms were implemented using the *FACTORIE* toolkit ([11]).

3.2   Results and Analysis

In the following all results were obtained by evaluating our approach on the two datasets using 10-fold cross validation. Classification performance was evaluated by the area under the *ROC*-curve (*AUC*) value, and the best accuracy achieved by the models. For the latter the focus lies on a high precision because it can indicate that the model has learned some characteristic path patterns which are common to at least a reasonable subset of positive training examples (e.g., Table 1).

Impact of Path Length: Table 2 compares the impact of different path lengths (up to 3 or 4) and feature types (*plain* or *LDA*). The table shows that the suggested approach can achieve an *AUC* up to 0.75 for the *may treat* and up to 0.8 for the *has target* relation. Especially for the *has target* relation we can observe high precisions up to 0.87 at reasonable recall levels around 0.6. With regards to the impact of the path length, the results show that using paths of length 4 does not improve the overall performance on the classification task. This could be due to the fact, that with increasing maximum length the number of additional informative paths gets lower while the total number of extracted

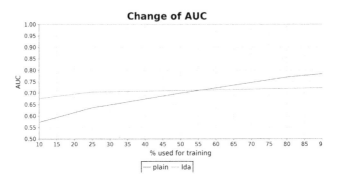

Fig. 2. Change of classification performance using different amounts of training data

paths gets exponentially bigger and so does the feature space. This can lead to overfitting of the model to the training data, because data is sparse compared to the huge feature space in these experiments.

Comparison of Feature Types: The impact of the different feature types, namely *plain* and *LDA*, cannot directly be inferred from the performances of the classifier on 10-fold cross validation shown in Table 2. In the *may treat* dataset the *LDA* encoding helps, in contrast to the *has target* dataset, which contains about double the amount of training examples. Therefore, in order to evaluate the impact of the different feature types, experiments with different amounts of training examples of the *has target* dataset were conducted. The results are presented in Figure 2.

The *plain* line (blue) shows that using one-of-N features depends highly on the amount of supplied training data, whereas the *lda* line (orange) shows that models trained on examples with *LDA* features do not. This shows the potential of encoding relations with *LDA*, as it transfers them into a much lower-dimensional, semantic space, which reduces the amount of necessary training data.

4   Conclusions

In this paper we have introduced a novel approach for relation discovery in the biomedical domain. The approach is based on the combination of information extracted from structured and unstructured data, and represented in a graph. The constructed graph allows for the easy integration of heterogeneous information and discovery of indirect connections between biomedical concepts. Given a biomedical relation and example pairs, graph paths are used to create feature vectors with which characteristic path patterns for this relation are learned. For the experimental evaluation of the approach we used two common biomedical relations; *has target* and *may treat*. The results are promising; primarily they show the feasibility of discovering relations using indirect connections between concepts. In addition they indicate that the suggested approach can discover the tested relations with an AUC of up to 0.8. Furthermore, the application of our approach in these two datasets suggests that it can be applied even when the data is sparse.

The experimental analysis also showed some limitations of the approach. First, the problem of incomplete knowledge in the biomedical domain. For example, the extraction of information from text does not take co-references into account. The same problem holds for the structured data sources, where the UMLS is missing some important relations, like *protein-to-protein* interactions, and the existing relations do not cover all currently known facts. Second, the erroneous annotation of the MEDLINE text with MetaMap, e.g., in the case of gene annotation. Finally, the approach does not consider currently the wider context of a statement extracted from an abstract. However, some important correlations between co-occurring pieces of information can be learned from the global context of entities, which constitutes one of the greatest advantages of the current approach. Towards our future work, we will focus in addressing the aforementioned problems, paying special attention to enriching the dependency paths with quantitative and qualitative information extracted from respective attributes that appear in the sentences together with the dependency paths.

References

1. Swanson, D.: Fish oil, raynaud's syndrome, and undiscovered public knowledge. Perspect. Bio. Med 30, 7–18 (1986)
2. Cohen, T., Schvaneveldt, R., Widdows, D.: Reflective random indexing and indirect inference: a scalable method for discovery of implicit connections. J. Biomed. Inform. 43(2), 240–256 (2010)
3. Frijters, R., van Vugt, M., Smeets, R., van Schaik, R.C., de Vlieg, J., Alkema, W.: Literature mining for the discovery of hidden connections between drugs, genes and diseases. PLoS Computational Biology 6(9) (2010)
4. Goertzel, B., Goertzel, I.F., Pinto, H., Ross, M., Heljakka, A., Pennachin, C.: Using dependency parsing and probabilistic inference to extract relationships between genes, proteins and malignancies implicit among multiple biomedical research abstracts. In: BioNLP, pp. 104–111 (2006)
5. Vizenor, L., Bodenreider, O., McCray, A.T.: Auditing associative relations across two knowledge sources. Journal of Biomedical Informatics 42(3), 426–439 (2009)
6. Lao, N., Subramanya, A., Pereira, F., Cohen, W.W.: Reading the web with learned syntactic-semantic inference rules. In: EMNLP-CoNLL, pp. 1017–1026 (2012)
7. Aronson, A.R.: Effective mapping of biomedical text to the UMLS Metathesaurus: the MetaMap program. In: AMIA Symposium, pp. 17–21 (2001)
8. Snow, R., Jurafsky, D., Ng, A.Y.: Learning syntactic patterns for automatic hypernym discovery. In: NIPS (2004)
9. Blei, D.M., Ng, A.Y., Jordan, M.I.: Latent dirichlet allocation. J. Mach. Learn. Res. 3, 993–1022 (2003)
10. Mimno, D.M., Hoffman, M.D., Blei, D.M.: Sparse stochastic inference for latent dirichlet allocation. In: ICML (2012)
11. McCallum, A., Schultz, K., Singh, S.: FACTORIE: Probabilistic programming via imperatively defined factor graphs. In: NIPS (2009)

Exploiting Semantics from Ontologies and Shared Annotations to Partition Linked Data

Guillermo Palma[1], Maria-Esther Vidal[1], Louiqa Raschid[2], and Andreas Thor[3]

[1] Universidad Simón Bolívar, Venezuela
[2] University of Maryland, USA
[3] University of Leipzig, Germany
{gpalma@,mvidal}@ldc.usb.ve, louiqa@umiacs.umd.edu,
thor@informatik.uni-leipzig.de

Abstract. Linked Open Data initiatives have made available a diversity of collections that domain experts have annotated with controlled vocabulary terms from ontologies. We identify annotation signatures of linked data that associate semantically similar concepts, where similarity is measured in terms of shared annotations and ontological relatedness. Formally, an annotation signature is a partition or clustering of the links that represent the relationships between shared annotations. A clustering algorithm named *AnnSigClustering* is proposed to generate annotation signatures. Evaluation results over drug and disease datasets demonstrate the effectiveness of using annotation signatures to identify patterns among entities in the same cluster of a signature.

1 Introduction

Ontologies are developed by domain experts to capture knowledge specific to some domain, and they have been widely adopted in the last decade. Simultaneously, Linked Open Data initiatives have made available a diversity of collections, and some of these datasets have been annotated by domain experts with controlled vocabulary (CV) terms from these ontologies. For example, the biomedical community has taken the lead in such activities; every model organism database has genes and proteins that are widely annotated with CV terms from the Gene Ontology (GO). The challenge is to explore these rich and complex annotated datasets, together with the domain semantics captured within ontologies, to discover patterns of annotations across multiple concepts that may lead to potential discoveries. For genes, these patterns may involve cross-genome functional annotations, e.g., combining the GO functional annotations of two model organisms such as Arabidopsis thaliana (a plant) and C. elegans (a nematode or worm), to predict new gene function or protein-protein interactions. As a first step to discovering complex annotation patterns, we define an *annotation signature* between a pair of scientific concepts, e.g., a pair of drugs or a pair of genes. The *annotation signature* builds upon the shared annotations or shared CV terms between the pair of concepts. The *annotation signature* is represented by N parts or clusters of ontologically related shared CV terms. For example, the *annotation signature* for a (drug, drug) pair will be a set

H. Galhardas and E. Rahm (Eds.): DILS 2014, LNBI 8574, pp. 120–127, 2014.

of N clusters, where clusters include links among ontologically related disease terms from NCIt.

Formally, given two sets S_1 and S_2 of concepts, e.g., drugs and targets, we represent the set of links between S_1 and S_2 as a bi-type information network BG [9], and our objective is to determine an *annotation signature* based on BG. We define the *Annotation Signature Partition* problem as the partitioning of the edges of BG into clusters such that the value of the aggregated cluster density is maximized. Values of density denote how close is the number of links in a cluster to the maximal number of edges between the nodes in the cluster. We develop *AnnSigClustering*, a clustering solution that implements a greedy iterative algorithm to cluster the edges in BG. Our research focuses on exploiting domain specific semantic knowledge. This includes both the ontology structure and relationship types between nodes of BG. *AnnSigClustering* is able to produce clusters of closely related terms that may be useful to the domain scientist. Further, the choice of specific relationship types allows to refine the clusters of CV terms in the *annotation signature*. We perform an extensive evaluation of the effectiveness of the *annotation signature* on the LinkedCT dataset of drugs and diseases from NCIt and their associations through the clinical trials. A team of experts performed a preliminary evaluation to determine if signatures of diseases were meaningful.

This paper is organized in five sections. Our approach and experimental results are presented in Section 2 and 3, respectively. Related work is summarized in Section 4, and conclusions and future work are outlined in Section 5.

2   Our Approach

Our proposed approach relies on structural knowledge encoded in an annotation graph represented using a bi-type information network as the one illustrated in Example 1. We use two taxonomic distance measures to compute relatedness of the ontological annotations that comprise the graph, i.e., to decide when pairs of diseases in the graph are similar in terms of the NCI Thesaurus where these terms have been defined.

Example 1. An antineoplastic agent is a substance that inhibits the maturation, growth or spread of tumor cells. Monoclonal antibodies that are also antineoplastic agents have become an important tool in cancer treatments. When used as a medication, the non-proprietary drug name ends in -mab. Scientists are interested in studying the relationships between drugs and the corresponding diseases; drugs are annotated with the NCIt terms that correspond to the conditions that have been tested for these drugs. Figure 1 illustrates `Brentuximab` vedotin and `Catumaxomab`, and some of their annotations. Each path between a pair of conditions, e.g., `Colorectal Carcinoma` and `Stage IV Rectal Cancer` through the NCIt is identified using red circles which represent CV terms from the NCIt. From Figure 1, we may conclude that the shared disease signature for this pair of drugs includes four clusters. The five terms `Colon Carcinoma`, `Colorectal Carcinoma`, `Rectal Carcinoma`, `Stage IV Rectal Cancer`, and `Rectal Carcinoma` form `Cluster1`. Similarly, `Cluster2` includes `Head` and `Neck Neoplasm`, `Oropharyngeal Neoplasm`, and `Thyroid Gland Neoplasm`.

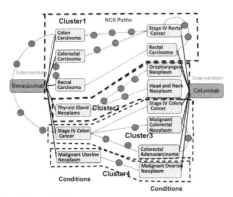

Fig. 1. Bi-type information network representing the annotations of Brentuximab vedotin and Cetumaxomab. Drugs are green rectangles; diseases are pink rectangles; NCIt terms are red circles. The annotation signature comprises four clusters: Cluster1, Cluster2, Cluster3, and Cluster4.

First, we consider the measure d_{tax} that captures the taxonomic distance between two vertices with respect to the depth of the common ancestor of these two vertices. d_{tax} assigns low(er) values of taxonomic distance to pairs of vertices that are: (1) at greater depth in the taxonomy, and (2) are closer to their lowest common ancestor. A value close to 0.0 means that the two vertices are close to the leaves and both are close to their lowest common ancestor. A value close to 1.0 represents that both vertices are general or that the lowest common ancestor is close to the root of the taxonomy. Then, $(1 - d_{tax})$ will be used as the similarity or *ontological relatedness* between nodes. The taxonomic distance metric d_{tax} is as follows, where *root* is the root node in the ontology; lca is the lowest common ancestor, and pl denotes path length:

$$d_{tax}(x, y) = \frac{pl(lca(x, y), x) + pl(lca(x, y), y)}{pl(root, x) + pl(root, y)} \quad (1)$$

We also define an extension of d_{tax} named d_{tax}^{str} that assigns low values of ontological similarity to pairs of terms where at least one of the terms is a general concept in the ontology. Let *MaxDepth_Ontology* represent the greatest depth in the ontology.

$$d_{tax}^{str}(A, B) = d_{tax}(A, B) * (1 - pFactor(A, B)) \quad (2)$$

$$pFactor(A, B) = \frac{\max(correctedDepth(A), correctedDepth(B))}{MaxDepth\_Ontology}$$

$$correctedDepth(X) = MaxDepth\_Ontology - Depth(X)$$

Our clustering algorithm implements a greedy iterative algorithm that heuristically assigns links to the clusters. Definition 1 outlines the conditions to be met for an edge to belong to the semantic 1-hop of a given edge in the bi-type information network.

Definition 1 (Semantic 1-Hop). *Given a bi-type information network BG=($A_i ∪ A_j$, WE), two distance metrics d_i and d_j for elements in A_i and A_j, respectively, and two real numbers $θ_i$ and $θ_j$ in the range [0.0:1.0]. The semantic 1-hop of an edge $e = (a, b)$ in WE, such that $a ∈ A_i$, and $b ∈ A_j$, s-1-hop($e, θ_i, θ_j, d_i, d_j$), is the set of all $e_h = (a_h, b_h)$ edges in WE and in the neighborhood of e that meet the following conditions:*

- a_h *and* a *are similar under* $θ_i$, *i.e.,* $d_i(a_h, a) ≤ θ_i$, *or*
- b_h *and* b *are similar under* $θ_j$, *i.e.,* $d_j(b_h, b) ≤ θ_j$.

Definition 2 (Cluster Density). *Given a bi-type information network BG=($A_i \cup A_j$, WE), d a distance metric between elements of A_i and A_j, and a subset p of WE, the cluster density of p corresponds to* $cDensity(p) = \frac{\sum_{e=(a,b)\in p} 1-d(a,b)}{|p|}$.

Definition 3 (The Annotation Signature Partition Problem (AnnSig)). *Given a bi-type information network BG=($A_i \cup A_j$, WE), d a distance metric between elements of A_i and A_j, and a real number θ in the range [0.0:1.0]. For each $a \in A_i$ and $b \in A_j$, if 1-d(a,b)> θ, then there is an edge e = (a, b) ∈ WE. For each e = (a, b) ∈ WE, label(e)= 1-d(a,b)). The AnnSig Partition Problem identifies a (minimal) partition P of WE s.t. the aggregate cluster density P* $AnnSig(P) = \frac{\sum_{p\in P}(cDensity(p))}{|P|}$ *is maximal.*

AnnSigClustering is a greedy iterative algorithm to solve the *Annotation Signature* Partition Problem. *AnnSigClustering* adds an edge to a cluster following a greedy heuristic to create clusters that maximize the cluster density. Given a bi-type information network $BG=(A_i \cup A_j, WE)$, two distance metrics d_i and d_j for elements in A_i and A_j, respectively, and two real numbers $θ_i$ and $θ_j$ in the range [0.0:1.0], *AnnSigClustering* orders edges in *WE* dynamically based on the number of different clusters assigned to the edges that are in the complement of *s-1-hop(e, $θ_i$, $θ_j$, d_i, d_j)*, i.e., the edges are chosen based on the degree of saturation on the partial clustering built so far. Only edges that are in the complement of the semantic 1-hop of the clustered edges are considered. Intuitively, selecting an edge with the maximum degree of saturation allows one to first cluster the edges with more restrictions; this is one for which there is a smaller set of potential cluster. Ties are broken based on the cardinality of the semantic 1-hop of the tied edges. The time complexity of *AnnSigClustering* is $O(|WE|^3)$. To illustrate the behavior of *AnnSigClustering*, let's consider the annotated graph in Figure 1. This graph can be partitioned into four groups of edges. Cluster1 includes the edges between Colon Carcinoma, Colorectal Carcinoma, and Rectal Carcinoma on the left with the terms Stage IV Rectal Cancer and Rectal Carcinoma on the right. Also, the edges from Thyroid Gland Neoplasm belong to Cluster2 , all the edges from Stage IV Colon Cancer are in Cluster3 , and the edge from Malignant Uterine Neoplasm to Malignant Ovarian Neoplasm is alone in Cluster4 .

3   Related Work

Graph data mining [4] covers a broad range of methods dealing with the identification of (sub)structures and patterns in graphs. Popular techniques include graph clustering, community detection, and cliques. The problem of a 1-to-1 weighted maximal bipartite match has been applied to many problems, e.g., semantic equivalence between two sentences and measuring similarity between shapes for object recognition[2]. These approaches clearly show the benefits of solving a matching problem to identify similarity between terms or concepts. Our research advances prior research in that we consider the relatedness of sets of annotations and identify a many-to-many bi-type match between links that relate similar concepts. A key element in finding patterns is identifying related concepts; we consider ontological relatedness. Similarity measures can be used to compute relatedness; we briefly describe some of the existing metrics. The first class of metrics are string-similarity[3]; they compare the names or labels of the concepts using string comparison functions based on edit distances or other functions that compare strings. This includes the Levenstein distance and Jaro-Winkler [5]. The next are path-similarity metrics that compute relatedness based on the paths that connect the concepts within some appropriate graph. Nodes in the paths can be all of the same abstract types (e.g., PathSim [8]) or they can be heterogeneous (HeteSim [7]). Furthermore, topological-similarity metrics extend the concept of path-similarity and they look at relationships within an ontology or taxonomy that is itself designed to capture relationships (e.g., d_{ps} [6] and d_{tax}[1]). We propose an approach that exploits ontological knowledge of scientific annotations to decide relatedness between annotated entities.

4   Evaluation

The goal of our evaluation is to validate if annotation signatures group together meaningful terms across shared annotations. Additionally, we evaluate the impact of the semantics encoded in the ontologies on the quality of the signature. We study an annotated dataset of twelve drugs that fall within the intersection of anti-neoplastic agents and monoclonal antibodies: Alemtuzumab, Bevacizumab, Brentuximab vedotin, Cetuximab, Catumaxomab, Edrecolomab, Gemtuzumab, Ipilimumab, Ofatumumab, Panitumumab, Rituximab, and Trastuzumab. The protocol to create the dataset is as follows: Each drug was used to retrieve a set of clinical trials in LinkedCT *circa* September 2011 (linkedct.org). Then each disease associated with each trial was linked to its corresponding term in the NCI Thesaurus version 12.05d; annotation was performed by NCIt experts. We relied on a team of experts to analyze the annotation signatures [1]. Our group of evaluators included two experts who develop databases and tools for the NCI Thesaurus, and two bioinformatics researchers with expertise on the NCIt and other biomedical ontologies.

Connectivity patterns within components provide insight into the ontological relatedness of the diseases. In Figure 2(a) Carcinoma on the left is connected to eight terms on the right. In Figure 2(b), Sarcoma on the left is connected to nine drugs on the right. Similarly, Breast Neoplasm on the right is connected to eight diseases on the left. None of the other drugs has more than one incident edge. In contrast, in Figure 2(c), we see a much more general many-to-many connection pattern between the diseases on the left and right. Finally, Figure 2(d) shows a more complex connectivity pattern where the terms are ontologically related but they are placed within three disconnected graphs. The four terms Diffuse Intrinsic Pontine Glioma, Spinal Cord Ependymoma, Carcinoma, and Squamous Cell Neoplasm form the most well connected component. An evaluation of patterns is being performed, and preliminary comments from the evaluators noted that while groups such as Figure 2(a) that included generic terms such as Carcinoma were valid, they did not convey useful information. In contract, groups in Figures 2(c) and (d), that had more specific terms and were more densely connected, having the potential to be more meaningful.

Additionally, we evaluate the impact of utilizing the ontology structure. Recall that d_{tax}^{str} extended the taxonomic distance metric d_{tax} to consider ontology structure. Fig-

---

[1] Results available at dynbigraph.appspot.com

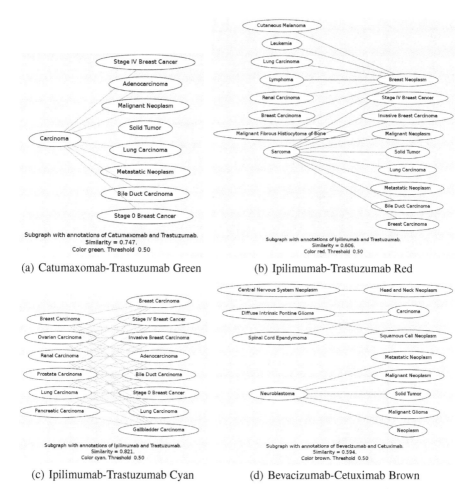

(a) Catumaxomab-Trastuzumab Green

(b) Ipilimumab-Trastuzumab Red

(c) Ipilimumab-Trastuzumab Cyan

(d) Bevacizumab-Cetuximab Brown

Fig. 2. Connectivity Patterns within Each Cluster for $\theta = 0.5$; we name the clusters with colors (a) Catumaxomab-Trastuzumab Green; (b) Ipilimumab-Trastuzumab Red; (c) Ipilimumab-Trastuzumab Cyan; (d) Bevacizumab-Cetuximab Brown

ure 3(a) illustrates an exemplar cluster of the annotations for the pair Trastuzumab and Bevacizumab produced by d_{tax}; the threshold $\theta = 0.50$. There are many shortcomings. First, it contains generic CV terms such as Adenocarcinoma and Carcinoma. Further, it is very large and many diverse and unrelated cancers are included. Figure 3(b) shows the result of applying the metric d_{tax}^{str} to exploit ontology structure. The large cluster was partitioned into smaller clusters. Many of the generic CV terms are no longer included and each smaller cluster includes more closely related CV terms. For example, one has a focus on breast cancer related terms, another has a focus on lung cancer, while a third combines terms related to pancreatic, renal, and colorectal cancers. This example illustrates benefits from using ontological knowledge to eliminate generic terms from the annotation signatures. Redundancy in patterns is reduced, and the modified annotation

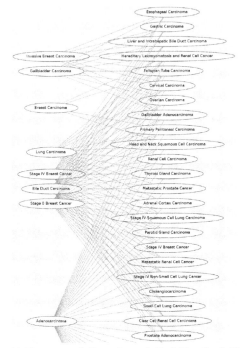

(a) Trastuzumab-Bevacizumab Cadeblue $\theta = 0.50$

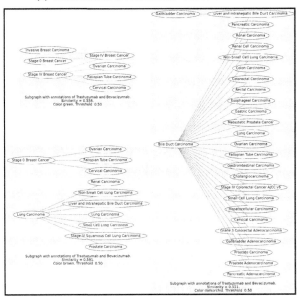

(b) Trastuzumab-Bevacizumab $\theta = 0.50$ using d_{tax}^{str}

Fig. 3. Enhancing Signatures with Semantics for $\theta = 0.50$. (a) Signature of Trastuzumab-Bevacizumab $\theta = 0.50$; Similarity d_{tax}-Figure has been truncated for readability.; (b) Three clusters of Trastuzumab-Bevacizumab $\theta = 0.50$ when generic terms are penalized using d_{tax}^{str}.

signatures are comprised of relationships between more specific terms, which according to the experts have the potential to be more meaningful.

5 Conclusions and Future Work

We have defined the *Annotation Signature* Partitioning problem and the *AnnSigClustering* algorithm to develop the components of a signature based on shared annotations and ontological relatedness. We empirically studied the effectiveness of *AnnSigClustering* to identify potential meaningful signatures of annotated concepts. Further, we have analyzed the effects of considering knowledge encoded in the ontologies used to annotate Linked Data. Our results suggest that the grouping capability of our approach is enhanced whenever the type of relationships are considered as well as when relationships with generic terms are eliminated. Our initial project objective was to validate correctness and utility of components in a signature. Nevertheless, in the future, we will also address performance and scalability. Additionally, we plan to conduct a deeper evaluation study with our collaborators, and thus determine the potential discovery capability of the approach. Finally, we plan to apply our techniques to other domains, e.g., to identify patterns of viral diseases.

References

1. Benik, J., Chang, C., Raschid, L., Vidal, M.-E., Palma, G., Thor, A.: Finding cross genome patterns in annotation graphs. In: Bodenreider, O., Rance, B. (eds.) DILS 2012. LNCS, vol. 7348, pp. 21–36. Springer, Heidelberg (2012)
2. Bhagwani, S., Satapathy, S., Karnick, H.: Semantic textual similarity using maximal weighted bipartite graph matching. In: Proceedings of the First Joint Conference on Lexical and Computational Semantics-Volume 1: Proceedings of the main conference and the shared task, and Volume 2: Proceedings of the Sixth International Workshop on Semantic Evaluation, pp. 579–585. Association for Computational Linguistics (2012)
3. Cohen, W.W., Ravikumar, P.D., Fienberg, S.E.: A comparison of string distance metrics for name-matching tasks. In: IIWeb, pp. 73–78 (2003)
4. Cook, D.J., Holder, L.B.: Mining graph data. Wiley-Blackwell (2007)
5. Jaro, M.A.: Probabilistic linkage of large public health data files. In: Statistics in Medicine, pp. 491–498 (1995)
6. Pekar, V., Staab, S.: Taxonomy learning - factoring the structure of a taxonomy into a semantic classification decision. In: COLING (2002)
7. Shi, C., Kong, X., Yu, P.S., Xie, S., Wu, B.: Relevance search in heterogeneous networks. In: EDBT, pp. 180–191 (2012)
8. Sun, Y., Han, J., Yan, X., Yu, P.S., Wu, T.: Pathsim: Meta path-based top-k similarity search in heterogeneous information networks. PVLDB 4(11), 992–1003 (2011)
9. Sun, Y., Han, J., Zhao, P., Yin, Z., Cheng, H., Wu, T.: Rankclus: integrating clustering with ranking for heterogeneous information network analysis. In: EDBT, pp. 565–576 (2009)

ConQuR-Bio: Consensus Ranking with Query Reformulation for Biological Data

Bryan Brancotte[1,2], Bastien Rance[4,5], Alain Denise[1,2,3],
and Sarah Cohen-Boulakia[1,2]

[1] Laboratoire de Recherche en Informatique (LRI), CNRS UMR 8623,
Université Paris-Sud, 91405 Orsay Cedex, France
[2] AMIB Group, INRIA Saclay Ile-de-France, France
[3] Institut de Génétique et de Microbiologie (IGM), CNRS UMR 8621,
Université Paris-Sud, France
[4] Biomedical Informatics and Public Health Department,
University Hospital Georges Pompidou, AP-HP, Paris, France
[5] INSERM Centre de Recherche des Cordeliers, team 22: Information Sciences to
support Personalized Medicine, Université Paris Descartes, Sorbonne Paris Cité,
Faculté de médecine, Paris, France

Abstract. This paper introduces ConQuR-Bio which aims at assisting
scientists when they query public biological databases. Various reformulations of the user query are generated using medical terminologies. Such
alternative reformulations are then used to rank the query results using
a new consensus ranking strategy. The originality of our approach thus
lies in using *consensus ranking* techniques within the context of *query
reformulation*. The ConQuR-Bio system is able to query the Entrez-
Gene NCBI database. Our experiments demonstrate the benefit of using
ConQuR-Bio compared to what is currently provided to users. ConQuR-
Bio is available to the bioinformatics community at
`http://conqur-bio.lri.fr`.

1   Introduction

In Biological research, findings are derived from the proper analysis of experiments which involves comparing at various scales new results obtained to existing
data. Over the last three decades, scientists have had to face with an avalanche
of data, of different kinds, and reported in a myriad of databases. Public biological databases thus contain more biological data than ever, all available to the
scientific community. Large amounts of data can be easily obtained using portals
such as Entrez NCBI[1] [14] daily used by the bioinformatics community by submitting *key-phrase queries* (list of keywords). However, properly querying such
portals is not as easy as one may think. Two very similar queries may provide
different sets of answers leading to the need for users to try various reformulations of their questions, considering synonymous terms, alternative spellings,
various levels of granularity in the concepts involved in their queries (making use
or not of the terminologies available such as MeSH [13] or SNOMED CT [16]).

---

[1] `http://www.ncbi.nlm.nih.gov/Entrez`

H. Galhardas and E. Rahm (Eds.): DILS 2014, LNBI 8574, pp. 128–142, 2014.
© Springer International Publishing Switzerland 2014

Results obtained should then be gathered, compared, and redundancies filtered out... Each set of results is ranked by the portal usually using the *relevance* as a ranking criteria (number of occurrences of the key-phrase in each piece of results instance). However, when several reformulations are considered, it is not clear how to rank the set of all the collected results, which may involve hundreds of elements. The expected ranking should be able to emphasize answers provided by various reformulations while putting less importance on elements classified as "good" by only a few.

The need for on-the-fly solutions both able to reformulate automatically queries exploiting the various terminologies available and rank answers provided to the user is thus of paramount importance.

In this paper, we introduce the ConQuR-Bio approach, which allows users to query public databases from NCBI while generating automatically all the possible reformulations and provides ranked answers using consensus ranking techniques.

The remainder of this paper is organized as follows. After a description of a set of use cases which have driven the design of our solution (Section 2), Section 3 introduces the architecture of our system. We present the original consensus ranking strategy we follow in Section 4. Section 5 introduces the interface and the main functionalities of the system we have implemented based on the ConQuR-Bio approach (available for use to the community at: `http://conqur-bio.lri.fr`). Section 6 provides the results obtained by ConQuR-Bio on several biological queries while Section 7 concludes the paper.

2   Use Cases

Our approach is based on one of the most popular tool for querying biological sources, namely, the Entrez portal [15] from the *National Center for Biotechnology Information* (NCBI). More specifically, the kind of queries we consider consists in searching the gene names associated to a given disease by consulting the EntrezGene database [14] and focusing answers to human genes. We describe here-after a set of four use cases that we want to consider.

Use Case 1 (equivalent reformulations): Let us consider the case of a single user interested in genes involved in the cervical cancer. To express her query, she may type *cervix cancer* in the search field of EntrezGene. As a result, 460 genes are obtained. Interestingly, her query could have been expressed in two other ways, namely using *cervical cancer* and *cancer of the cervix*, leading respectively to 20 and 2 results, with 9 new genes of interest obtained (compared to the original query).

Use Case 2 (abbreviations): Another use case is related to the use of abbreviations in queries. Consider searching for genes associated to *Attention deficit hyperactivity disorders* also known as ADHD. While the full name of the disease returns 144 genes, its abbreviation provides 109 genes with only 74 in common.

Use Case 3 (lexical-based reformulation): Another typical use case consists in considering two users, one from the US the other from the UK, searching for *tumor suppressor genes* associated to the *breast cancer*. While the first one enters *breast cancer tumor suppressor*, the other enters *breast cancer tumour suppressor*. This orthographic variation leads to huge differences when querying the EntrezGene database: 681 genes are returned with *tumor* and 291 with *tumour*, and only 246 genes are common to both queries.

Use Case 4 (narrower-term-based reformulation): In a last use case, we consider the case of diseases presenting a variety of subtypes (usually corresponding to multiple phenotypes or a gradient of phenotypes associated with the disease). For example, when the *colorectal cancer* is hereditary and without polyposis it can be described by various names, including *Hereditary Nonpolyposis Colon Cancer*, also known as *Lynch syndrome*. Interestingly, querying the EntrezGene database with *Hereditary Nonpolyposis Colon Cancer*, and *Lynch syndrome*, allows to respectively find 1, and 6 genes which were not found when typing *colorectal cancer*.

From these use cases, the need for automatic reformulation of queries appears clearly as a necessity. Even more importantly, faced with the high number of answers obtained as result of each query (especially when several reformulations are considered), users should be guided in the order to which consider results. The originality of our approach lies in considering alternative reformulations of the user query and exploiting these reformulations to rank the results by order of interest (roughly, genes obtained by a large number of reformulations should be ranked before genes returned by only a few).

3   The ConQuR-Bio Approach

In this section, we introduce ConQuR-Bio (Consensus ranking with Query Reformulation for Biological data) which aims at helping users finding genes associated to a given disease by considering various reformulations of each user query and exploiting such reformulations to rank the list of results. More precisely, our approach takes in several input rankings (several lists of genes, each provided by one reformulation) and outputs a *consensus ranking*, that is, a unified list considering all the input data ordered such that the disagreements between the list and the input rankings are minimized.

In the following, the main architecture of our approach is first presented, then two focuses are given, on the *reformulation module* and *queries generator module*.

3.1   General Architecture

The standard use of ConQuR-Bio consists in the user providing a *key-phrase k* (i.e., a list of keywords). The key-phrase is sent (arrow ☐1 in Figure 1) to the *Reformulation Module* which decomposes k into a list T of terms and leverage various terminologies to generate the set S of synonyms (cf 3.2). S is then trans-

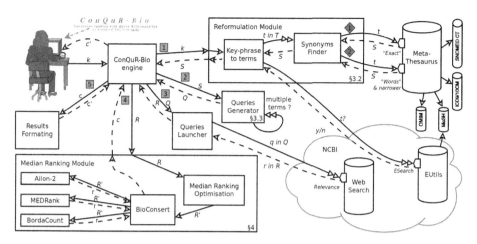

Fig. 1. Architecture of ConQuR-Bio. Solid arrows represent requests and dotted arrows responses. Two headed arrows represent possibly iterative requests. When several actions have to be done successively, their are numbered with a squared number. When alternative actions can be done, actions are represented with a diamonded number.

mitted (through arrow 2) to the *Queries Generator* to be expressed as a set Q of queries (cf 3.3). Q are run online (arrow 3) on the selected search engine (in our case, the NCBI web search engine for EntrezGene which provides sets of results ranked by *relevance*). When all the ranked results R of queries Q have been collected, they are sent 4 to the *Median Ranking Module* which is in charge of computing a unique consensus ranking, providing an ordering of all the answers (cf 4). Finally, 5 the *Results Formatting* module enriches the ranking of gene identifiers with names and descriptions.

A few parameters may be tuned by users, such as the selection of the species of interest (by default, *Human*) or the "Search deeper" option in which the *Reformulation Module* intends to find more reformulations for each term (details in 3.2). A default configuration is provided.

3.2   Reformulation Module

One of the two main modules of ConQuR-Bio is the *Reformulation Module*. It takes the user key-phrase as input, splits it into a list of terms and returns sets of reformulations for each term. The *Reformulation Module* leverages several medical terminologies within the UMLS® [3]. The terminologies are described here-after followed by the presentation of the process used to exploit such terminologies in ConQuR-Bio.

Terminologies Used. ConQuR-Bio makes use of the Unified Medical Language System® (UMLS)[2], a terminology integration system developed at the U.S. Na-

---

[2] Version 2013AB of the UMLS is used in the current version of ConQuR-Bio and for the evaluation we provide in the next section

tional Library of Medicine (NLM). ConQuR-Bio uses the UMLS API to interact with the Metathesaurus® integrating more than 160 medical vocabularies. Our approach particularly benefits from the use of five terminologies covering a wide range of biomedical domains: (i) MeSH [13], developed at the U.S. NLM and designed for indexing PubMed; (ii) SNOMED CT [16], a worldwide used clinical terminology often used as a core for Electronic Health Records; (iii and iv) The two latest versions of the International Classification of Diseases (ICD 9 CM and ICD 10 CM), developed by the World Health Organization and used in hospitals; (v) The Online Mendelian Inheritance in Man (OMIM), cataloging all known genetic diseases in the human genome. Each UMLS concept is categorized with at least one *Semantic Type* (out of 150+) from the Semantic Network. The UMLS also provides a broad categorization of Semantic Types into 15 *Semantic Groups* (including Disorders). Using the Metathesaurus allows to access synonymous terms from the terminologies.

From Key-Phrase to MeSH Terms. MeSH being de facto a *lingua franca* for biomedical literature querying, ConQuR-Bio starts with finding the largest recognized MeSH terms in the key-phrase provided by the user. More precisely, the key-phrase is decomposed into a list of terms where each term belongs to one terminology, but no concatenation of two or more consecutive terms belongs to any terminology. For example, the query "breast cancer oncogene" matches four MeSH terms "breast" "cancer", "oncogene" but also "breast cancer". The key-phrase is thus decomposed into the two terms "breast cancer" and "oncogene".

Reformulation Modes. Once the MeSH terms in the query have been identified, ConQuR-Bio may follow two modes to find reformulated terms, leveraging the UMLS to identify synonyms of (◆) the MeSH terms from the original query (default search mode), or (◆) more precise (i.e. narrower) terms and their synonyms. In any case, alternative formulations of the query are generated. When only one reformulation is returned by the default search mode (◆) (meaning that the term is recognized but has no synonym) then the second mode (◆) (using narrower terms and their synonyms) is used. The second mode is also used in complement of the first mode when the *search deeper mode* is enabled.

Identifying Synonyms (Arrow (◆)). The default mode uses the UMLS API *exact match* search strategy to find UMLS concepts associated with each term. From these concepts, we extract all the synonymous terms from SNOMED CT, ICD9, ICD10 and MeSH, associated with this UMLS concept. For example, the term *cervix carcinoma* is mapped to the UMLS concept C0302592. This concept includes several synonyms, including *Cancer of cervix* (from SNOMED CT) and *Uterine Cervical Cancer* (from MeSH).

Identifying Narrower Terms (Arrow (◆)). This alternative mode provides reformulations using narrower terms (in the sense of the organization of the hierarchy), which are thus more precise terms than the terms used in the original query.

Synonyms of the narrower terms are also exploited. This mode corresponds to use UMLS API *word* search strategy. For example, using the "word" search strategy from with the term *Long QT syndrome* (UMLS concept C0023976) allows to identify several narrower concepts, including *Long QT syndrome type 1* (UMLS concept C0035828, for which *Romano-Ward syndrome* is a synonym).

Semantic Filtering. As searched terms are all expected to be diseases, only mappings to concepts from the UMLS semantic group *Disorders* are considered.

3.3   Queries Generator Module

The *Queries generator module* produces queries from the synonyms found for the terms identified in the user's key-phrase by the *Reformulation Module* (see 3.2). When the key-phrase has been split into multiple terms, we consider the Cartesian product of the reformulations of each term. Considering a key-phrase k composed of two terms a and b such as $k = "a\ b"$ and a, resp. b, is reformulated into $\{a, a'\}$, resp. $\{b, b'\}$. This module generates queries to search for "$a\ b$", "$a'\ b$", "$a\ b'$", "$a'\ b'$".

4   The Median Ranking Module

In this section we present the *Median Ranking module*, one of the major modules of ConQuR-Bio which provides a unique ranking to the user. This module takes in lists of elements (here, lists of genes), each list being obtained by a given reformulation. It outputs a *consensus ranking*, that is, a list of all the elements present in the inputs, ordered such that the disagreements between the consensus and the input rankings is minimized.

In the following, we first define the median ranking problem; we then show that a new metric is needed for our approach, and, for this purpose, we define a pseudometric for comparing rankings. Finally, we describe the heuristic that we have developed and tuned to compute consensus ranking, driven by the need to provide an on-the-fly solution.

4.1   The Median Ranking Problem

Starting with multiple rankings called *input rankings*, the MEDIAN RANKING PROBLEM consists in finding one *ranking* able to minimize the distance to the input rankings. When the Kendall-τ distance is considered [12], the input rankings must be over the same elements and the problem of finding an optimal solution is known to be NP-Hard when more than 3 rankings are considered [9]. Polynomial-time approximation algorithms and heuristics have thus been proposed (*e.g.* [11,1]). In this paper, we will call *consensus* the solutions proposed by consensus algorithms (including heuristics or approximation algorithms), while we will use the term *median rankings* to denote optimal solutions.

We consider here rankings with ties, that is, rankings where some elements may be grouped into one bucket and may thus not been compared to each others. More precisely, each bucket contains at least one element, and two elements have a different rank iff they are in two different buckets. For instance, in the ranking $r = [\{B, A\}, \{C\}, \{D\}]$, the elements A and B are tied in a bucket and thus equally good, they are also better than C and D, and C is better than D.

As underlined in the use cases introduced in section 2, two reformulations may not necessarily provide the same sets of data (i.e., sets of genes obtained may be different from one reformulation to another). Unifying the data sets taken as input is then the first step to achieve to compute the corresponding consensus ranking. ConQuR-Bio makes use of the *unification process* introduced by [7] to consider input rankings over different sets of elements. This treatment adds a single bucket at the end of each ranking and places in this bucket all the elements that appear in other rankings but not in the current one. We call such buckets *unifying buckets*. For example, consider $r' = [\{C\}, \{E\}]$ and the ranking r introduced above. The unifying process provides the two unified input rankings: $r'_{unified} = [\{C\}, \{E\}, \{A, B, D\}_u]$ and $r_{unified} = [\{B, A\}, \{C\}, \{D\}, \{E\}_u]$, leading to two input rankings over the same sets of elements (A to E). Note that unified buckets are suffixed: $\{...\}_u$.

When considering ranking with ties, the distance used in the median ranking problem is the generalized Kendall-τ distance [11,7] defined as follows:

Definition 1. *Let r and c be two ranking with ties over n elements, c being a consensus. Let $r[i]$ be the rank of i in ranking r. The generalized Kendall-τ distance is:*

$$K^{(p)}(r, c) = \#\{(i, j) : r[i] < r[j] \text{ and } c[i] > c[j] \text{ or}$$
$$r[i] > r[j] \text{ and } c[i] < c[j]\}$$
$$+ p * \#\{(i, j) : r[i] \neq r[j] \text{ and } c[i] = c[j] \text{ or}$$
$$r[i] = r[j] \text{ and } c[i] \neq c[j]\} \qquad \text{where } 0 < p \leq 1$$

This distance counts 1 for each pair of elements when their order is inverted, and counts p when two elements are tied in one ranking and not in the other. The distance between a consensus c and a set of input rankings R is the sum of the distances between c and the rankings in R: $K^{(p)}(R, c) = \sum_{r \in R} K^{(p)}(r, c)$. A *median* of a set of input rankings is defined as follows:

Definition 2. *Let $\mathcal{R}$ be the set of all rankings with ties over n elements, and let $R \subseteq \mathcal{R}$ be a set of rankings. A ranking c^* is called a median ranking of R iff:*

$$K^{(p)}(R, c^*) \leq K^{(p)}(R, r), \forall r \in \mathcal{R};$$

Example 1. Let us consider the set of input rankings $R = \{r_1, r_2, r_3\}$ where $r_1 = r_2 = [\{A\}, \{D\}, \{B, C\}_u]$, $r_3 = [\{B\}, \{A, D\}, \{C\}]$. The median ranking is $c^* = [\{A\}, \{D\}, \{B, C\}]$. The disagreements are: the order inversion of B-A and B-D (+2) plus A-D untying (+p) plus B-C tying (+p) thus $K^{(p)}(R, c^*) = 2 + 2p$.

4.2 A New Pseudometric to Compare Rankings

The intuition behind the need for a new metric can be illustrated on the above example. Two points should be emphasized. First, elements A and D are tied in r_3 because the search engine ranked them at the same position, they thus should be considered as equally relevant. Second, elements B and C are tied in r_1 and r_2 due to the unification process, contrary to the previous situation, no search engine has ever indicated any rank between such two elements (neither one before the other, nor both at the same position).

The generalized Kendall-τ distance does not allow to make a distinction between elements tied in an unification bucket from those tied in a classical one. A new metric taking into account the nature of buckets has thus to be defined. In particular, the metric should consider true disagreements between elements ranked by several reformulations while not penalizing any difference between the relative positions of elements present in the unifying buckets: our aim is to consider that untying elements from the unifying bucket has no cost.

Definition 3. *Let r and c be two rankings with ties over n elements. Let $r[i]$ be the rank of i in ranking r. Let $unif(r)$ denote the unification bucket of r. $(unif(r) = \emptyset$ if r has no unification bucket.) Let us define $\mathcal{M}(r,c)$ as follows:*

$$\mathcal{M}(r,c) = \#\{(i,j) : r[i] < r[j] \text{ and } c[i] > c[j] \text{ or}$$
$$r[i] > r[j] \text{ and } c[i] < c[j]\}$$
$$+p\#\{(i,j) : r[i] \neq r[j] \text{ and } c[i] = c[j] \text{ and } i \notin unif(c) \text{ or}$$
$$r[i] = r[j] \text{ and } c[i] \neq c[j] \text{ and } j \notin unif(r)\}$$

Clearly $\mathcal{M}$ is not a distance as it may not be always possible to distinguish two different rankings: $\mathcal{M}([\{A\}, \{B\}], [\{A, B\}_u]) = 0$. However, it is a pseudometric [17] as the symmetry and triangular inequality properties are respected, and any element has a metric at zero compared to itself: $\mathcal{M}(r,r) = 0$. Similarly to the generalized Kendall-τ distance, when considering a consensus c and a set of input rankings R: $\mathcal{M}(R,c) = \sum_{r \in R} \mathcal{M}(r,c)$.

Example 2. Let us consider a set of input rankings $R = \{r_1, r_2, r_3\}$ where $r_1 = r_2 = [\{A\}, \{D\}, \{B, C\}_u], r_3 = [\{B\}, \{A, D\}, \{C\}]$. Under the generalized Kendall-τ distance, the median ranking is $c = [\{A\}, \{D\}, \{B, C\}]$ (cf. *Example 1*) while under the pseudometric $\mathcal{M}$ the median ranking is $c' = [\{A\}, \{D\}, \{B\}, \{C\}]$ as $\mathcal{M}(R,c) = 2 + p > \mathcal{M}(R,c') = 2$ (note that $K^{(p)}(R,c') = 2 + 3p$). From a user perspective, c' is a better median than c as it still promotes A and D, but also makes use of information provided by r_3 such as the fact that B is more relevant than C.

Other strategies have been developed in [9] in order to deal with sets of rankings which are not necessarily over the same elements: the *induced* Kendall-τ distance allows to compare a ranking c over all elements with a ranking r over a subset of these elements. The idea is to consider the projection of c onto r, by removing from c all elements that are missing in r. However, this distance is not relevant for our purpose as it does not allow to consider missing elements as being less relevant than the returned ones (the missing elements of r are completely removed from c and thus do not contribute to any (dis)agreement).

4.3   Median Ranking in the Context of Query Reformulations

BioConsert [7] is an heuristic designed in the context of biological data and considers a distance between rankings with ties. It uses each input ranking as starting point, and refines them by iteratively applying two edit operators (moving an element to an existing/new bucket) as long as the distance between the current consensus obtained and the input rankings is reduced. Finally, it returns the best consensus computed. Our approach differs from [7] by using the pseudometric $\mathcal{M}$, presented in §4.2, instead of the generalized Kendall-τ distance. $\mathcal{M}$ is parametrized by $0 < p \leq 1$ which expresses the importance of tying and untying elements. In our setting, tying and untying elements should be penalized while when two elements have the same number of rankings placing one element before and after the other, the two elements should be tied. As a consequence, we have set $p = 0.5$ in ConQuR-Bio.

Tuning BioConsert. ConQuR-Bio is an on-the-fly system which intends to quickly provide a consensus ranking from the reformulations obtained. To do so, it requires to have a fast and good algorithm to produce the *consensus of answers*. The time complexity of BioConsert depends, among other parameters, on the number of input rankings m. In order to speed up the computation, we consider a smaller and constant amount of rankings to start the algorithm (and not all input rankings as in [7]). More precisely, we selected three state-of-the-art algorithms: BordaCount [4], MEDRank [10], and Ailon's 2-approximation [1] which do not provide as good results as BioConsert, but provide solution in at most complexities of $nm \, log(nm)$, where n is the number of elements to be ranked. Experiments (not shown here) performed to compare this new strategy to the default strategy of BioConsert show that the time to compute a consensus is reduced up to one hundred times while the quality of the results is not significantly altered.

5   The ConQuR-Bio System

The main interface of ConQuR-Bio is provided in Figure 2 and composed of three areas, the query area (top left panel), the running and progression details (top right panel), and the results (bottom).

In the query area, the key-phrase provided by the user is split into MeSH terms on-the-fly (cf. 3.2) and displayed into colored boxes next to the key-phrase field. Colors indicate different status for a term: green when the term is recognized as a MeSH term, red when the term is not recognized, and orange when the term is matched with an existing MeSH term while the spelling is different. In addition to the orange semantics, when a term is matched with an alternative spelling, a check mark allows the user to accept the correction and update the key-phrase field, while a cross mark forces the system to use the given spelling. Several options are made available to the user, and are by default hidden. They can be displayed/hidden by clicking on "[+]"/"[-]" like in Figure 2). Options are the

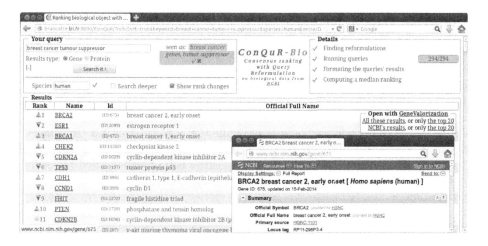

Fig. 2. ConQuR-Bio interface and the window open after clicking on BRCA2

species considered, the "Search deeper" mode which allows to use reformulations with narrower terms (cf. ◆ in 3.2), and the type of biological object ranked.

The results area presents a ranking (with ties) of genes with their official descriptions as it can be found when browsing the NCBI website. Each gene is linked to its associated page in the NCBI Website, allowing the user to navigate in a familiar environment. Close to the rank of each gene, a symbol (hidden in the default mode) allows users to know whether the rank of the gene is raised (▲), equal (=), lowered (▼), or new ( ) in ConQuR-Bio compared to the results returned in the NCBI ranking.

Another interesting feature is the ability of ConQuR-Bio to provide users with information on the number of publications associated with each gene returned. This functionality is obtained by calling the GeneValorization[6] tool able to quickly browse PubMed.

6   Results on Medical Queries

We have tested our approach over a set of queries collected from collaborators of the *Institut Curie (France)* and the *Children's Hospital of Philadelphia (PA, USA)* and linked to their respective fields of expertise. The results presented considered 9 diseases: 7 cancers (*bladder, breast, cervical, colorectal, neuroblastoma, prostate, retinoblastoma*), one heart disease (the *Long QT Syndrome*), and one psychiatric disorder (the *attention deficit (with) hyperactivity disorder*). For cancers, we searched for information on the name of the cancer while also using additional words (and reformulations of such words) to refine the query, namely *tumor suppressor* and *oncogene*. The exact list of words used are shown in Figure 3.

Evaluating such an approach is a difficult task as we face the users' perception of the results. We have chosen to consider three criteria of evaluation, focusing on the 20 first results returned for each key-phrase (top-20). The first criterion is based on *Gold Standards* and compares the results obtained to the list of expected genes according to our experts. We classically use the area under the ROC curve [5] in this series of experiments. The next two criteria are bibliometrics ones: the second criterion is the number of publications associated with each gene of the list and the key-phrase while the last criterion is a "freshness" indicator, measuring the average number of days since such an article has been published. The assumptions behind such measures is that well-studied genes are more likely to be relevant and experts can be interested in the latest, up-to-date, information.

6.1   Using Expertise

We constructed with our clinician collaborators the list l_d of the most relevant genes known to be associated with each disease d. The "goodness" of a consensus ranking c_d provided by ConQuR-Bio thus relies on the presence of elements of l_d in the top-ranked elements of c_d. In order to compare the results returned by ConQuR-Bio and the EntrezGene NCBI Web search engine with respect to *Gold Standards*, we used the Area Under the ROC Curve [5] (ROC standing for *Receiver Operating Characteristic*) or *AUC* (closely related to precision and recall measures [5]). The AUC aims at differentiating the presence of expected data versus non expected data, taking into account the place of pieces of data (roughly, placing expected data before unexpected data increases the score of the AUC). AUC provides numbers ranged in $[0, 1]$, 1 being the highest score.

In Figure 3, we plot AUCs for the top-20 first results obtained for each key-phrases with both NCBI search engine and ConQuR-Bio. Globally, using ConQuR-Bio compared to NCBI allows to increase in average the AUC of 44.24%. More precisely, four points deserve attention.

First, when focusing on single term key-phrases (i.e., considering the name of the disease only without adding *oncogene* or *tumo[u]r suppressor*, corresponding to Figure 3.a and all use cases), ConQuR-Bio returns better results than the NCBI in 88.89% of the cases and always provides as good results as the NCBI. The average AUC is increased of 58.52% with ConQuR-Bio compared to NCBI.

Second, multi-term key-phrases (Fig 3.b,c (use case 3)) have an AUC increased of 37.70% in average when using ConQuR-Bio compared to NCBI. This relatively less good results (37% vs. 58% of improvement) is actually due to the fact that the term *oncogene* has, in addition, one reformulation (*gene transforming*) less interesting (considered as "too vague" by our experts) than others.

Third, considering *ADHD* and its unabbreviated name (use case 2), the AUC is drastically increased using ConQuR-Bio. Also, as expected the complete name and its abbreviation have different AUCs with the NCBI while remaining the same with ConQuR-Bio (since all the reformulations are considered). In the same spirit, lexical variations around the *cervical cancer tumor suppressor* (Fig 3.b) show the importance of taking into account all lexical and orthographic variations: ConQuR-Bio returns identical results for the four variants with an AUC of 0.53 while NCBI results have systematically inferior and variable AUCs.

Finally, there were a few key-phrases, namely *colorectal cancer* and *neuroblastoma*, for which only plural reformulations were actually available (no actual synonyms available). The results obtained for such queries are then less impressive than in the previous cases while some of their respective AUCs are still increased compared to NCBI.

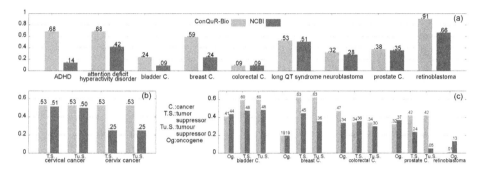

Fig. 3. The Area under the ROC curve (AUC) for the 20 first genes returned by ConQuR-Bio and the NCBI WebSearch for (a) Single-term key-phrases, (b) lexical variation around *cervix cancer tumor suppressor*, and (c) the remaining key-phrases.

Our experiments have shown that all the reformulations associated to use cases 1, 2, 3 were taken into account and that using our approach based on consensus ranking systematically improved the answers provided to the user. However, we have not yet provided specific information on the use case 4 which made use of lexical narrower terms. Two points should thus be mentioned.

First, interestingly, narrower terms have actually automatically been exploited in the previous results for the *long QT syndrome* as this term did not have any synonym. Specific forms of the disease, such as the *Romano Ward Syndrome*, raise the AUC from 0.51 to 0.53.

Second, the use of narrower terms can be done manually by selecting the "search deeper" option. Back to the example illustrating the use case 4, using narrower terms drastically change the results: among the 11 genes provided by our experts as being very relevant for *colorectal cancer*, only 2 are in the top-20 results of the NCBI (AUC=0.09) while 6 are in the ConQuR-Bio first 20 answers (AUC=0.43).

A last point that deserves attention is the time taken by ConQuR-Bio to provide answers: While the NCBI search engine provides a ranking in at most $2s$, ConQuR-Bio takes $41s$ in average for the 9 single term key-phrases listed in Figure 3.a. This difference lies in the fact that the average number of synonyms retrieved by ConQuR-Bio (and thus the average number of queries to be answered and which elements should be ranked) is 17.

6.2   Using the Number of Publications

The second measure considers the top-20 genes obtained and sums the number of publications co-citing each gene name and the query key-phrase. As an example, the numbers of publications associated with the top-20 first genes returned for *retinoblastoma* by the NCBI and ConQuR-Bio are represented in Figure 4. It clearly shows that the top-20 genes provided by ConQuR-Bio are associated to more publications than the top-20 genes provided by NCBI.

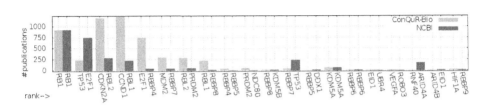

Fig. 4. #publications for each of the 20 first ranked genes for *retinoblastoma*

More generally, over the 28 key-phrases studied, 25 provide more (or, in 2 situation equal) publications than the NCBI. Overall in average, ConQuR-Bio returns top-20 results associated with 56% more publications.

6.3   Using Publication Freshness

While the number of publications is one important factor for determining the level of interest associated to a result, another complementary factor is the freshness of the associated publications (i.e. how recently studies based on a given gene have been published). The measure we consider in this subsection computes the average number of days since the last publication co-citing the gene name and the key-phrase has been published.

Over the 28 key-phrases studied, and when considering the top-20 genes, ConQuR-Bio returns genes with fresher results for 22 of them. In average, the top-20 genes returned by ConQuR-Bio have one associated article which was published within 25% less days that the NCBI ones.

7   Discussion

With ConQuR-Bio, we made the connection between the *query expansion* field and the *median ranking* field. We leveraged terminologies integration in the UMLS system (an approach and system shown to be effective [8]) to propose reformulations. From two UMLS search modes, we provided reformulations based on MeSH terms identified in the users key-phrases. To generate a consensus answer to the user emphasizing the agreements between the reformulations, we backed its computation on a new pseudometric, extending the state-of-the-art generalized Kendall-τ distance. With this new pseudometric, we adapted and combined several median ranking algorithms, allowing the system to quickly compute a consensus. We compared our approach to the main portal used to browse gene-centric biological data, namely the EntrezGene database from the NCBI website and its ranking function based on relevance. We showed that when measuring the presence and order of expected results (based on Gold standards), ConQuR-Bio outperforms the NCBI with an AUC increased of 69.30%. When focusing on biometrics indicators and compared to the NCBI relevance sorting, ConQuR-Bio returned genes associated with 56% more publications, published in 25% less days. Last but not least, we made the system available and free to use at `http://conqur-bio.lri.fr` as a website.

We now provide a discussion and perspectives considering the various steps of our approach.

ConQuR-Bio starts with identifying MeSH terms from key-phrases. We have currently chosen to follow a greedy (and naive) process enabling a very fast answer rate, compatible with the on-the-fly feature of our approach. This strategy is entirely satisfactory on evaluated key-phrases. Future work will explore the detection of concepts from the users key-phrases by deploying concept recognition software such as MetaMap [2] or BioAnnotator, enabling advanced reformulation options (e.g. different levels of granularity). Providing results in a few seconds while augmenting their overall quality will be the most challenging point.

The reformulation module plays a major role in the quality of the results. This module is based on two components: the set of terminologies used and the way such terminologies are queried and exploited.

As for the terminologies, we currently use terminology sources from the UMLS which allowed us to have manageable and relevant amounts of reformulations. Ongoing work includes selecting a larger and customizable number of sources from the main two biological terminology integration systems (namely, the UMLS and the BioPortal [18]) to cover a broader scope of biological domains. To cope with the possibly too broad aspect of reformulations, we plan to allow (experienced) users to select the reformulations to be or not to be used by our system.

As for the way terminologies are exploited, in our current version, the "search deeper" mode provides narrower reformulations. However, work still have to be done as the semantics of this mode is very permissive and does not exploit the hierarchical feature of the links between concepts. The UMLS system provides typed links for broader and narrower concepts unified between terminologies, and their adequacy should be evaluated. Ongoing work consists in exploiting the hierarchical relations from the sources to improve the detection of concepts and their synonyms.

References

1. Ailon, N.: Aggregation of Partial Rankings, p-Ratings and Top-m Lists. Algorithmica 57, 284–300 (2010)
2. Aronson, A.R.: Effective mapping of biomedical text to the umls metathesaurus: the metamap program. In: Proceedings of the AMIA Symposium, p. 17. American Medical Informatics Association (2001)
3. Bodenreider, O.: The unified medical language system (umls): integrating biomedical terminology. Nucleic Acids Research 32(suppl. 1), D267–D270 (2004)
4. de Borda, J.C.: Mémoire sur les élection au scrutin. Histoire de l'academie royal des sciences, 657–664 (1781)
5. Bradley, A.P.: The use of the area under the roc curve in the evaluation of machine learning algorithms. Pattern Recognition 30, 1145–1159 (1997)
6. Brancotte, B., Biton, A., Bernard-Pierrot, I., Radvanyi, F., Reyal, F., Cohen-Boulakia, S.: Gene List significance at-a-glance with GeneValorization. Bioinformatics 27(8), 1187–1189 (2011)
7. Cohen-Boulakia, S., Denise, A., Hamel, S.: Using Medians to Generate Consensus Rankings for Biological Data. In: Bayard Cushing, J., French, J., Bowers, S. (eds.) SSDBM 2011. LNCS, vol. 6809, pp. 73–90. Springer, Heidelberg (2011)
8. Demner-Fushman, D., Abhyankar, S., Jimeno-Yepes, A., Loane, R.F., Rance, B., Lang, F.-M., Ide, N.C., Apostolova, E., Aronson, A.R.: A knowledge-based approach to medical records retrieval. TREC (2011)
9. Dwork, C., Kumar, R., Naor, M., Sivakumar, D.: Rank aggregation methods for the web. In: Proceedings of the 10th World Widw Web Conference, pp. 613–622. ACM, New York (2001)
10. Fagin, R., Kumar, R., Sivakumar, D.: Efficient similarity search and classification via rank aggregation. In: Proceedings of the 2003 ACM SIGMOD International Conference on Management of Data, pp. 301–312. ACM (2003)
11. Fagin, R., Kumar, R., Mahdian, M., Sivakumar, D., Vee, E.: Comparing and aggregating rankings with ties. In: Proceedings of the Twenty-Third ACM SIGMOD-SIGACT-SIGART Symposium on Principles of Database Systems, PODS 2004, pp. 47–58. ACM, New York (2004)
12. Kendall, M.: A new measure of rank correlation. Biometrika 30, 81–89 (1938)
13. Carolyn, E.: Lipscomb. Medical subject headings (mesh). Bulletin of the Medical Library Association 88(3), 265 (2000)
14. Maglott, D., Ostell, J., Pruitt, K.D., Tatusova, T.: Entrez gene: gene-centered information at ncbi. Nucleic Acids Research 39(sp.1), D52–D57 (2011)
15. Sayers, E.W., Barrett, T., Benson, D.A., Bolton, E., Bryant, S.H., Canese, K., Chetvernin, V., Church, D.M., DiCuccio, M., Federhen, S., et al.: Database resources of the national center for biotechnology information. Nucleic Acids Research 39(suppl. 1), D38–D51 (2011)
16. Stearns, M.Q., Price, C., Spackman, K.A., Wang, A.Y.: Snomed clinical terms: overview of the development process and project status. In: Proceedings of the AMIA Symposium, p. 662 (2001)
17. Steen, L.A., Seebach, A., Steen, L.A.: Counterexamples in topology. Springer (1978)
18. Whetzel, P.L., Noy, N.F., Shah, N.H., Alexander, P.R., Nyulas, C., Tudorache, T., Musen, M.A.: Bioportal: enhanced functionality via new web services from the national center for biomedical ontology to access and use ontologies in software applications. Nucleic Acids Research 39(suppl. 2), D541–D545 (2011)

An Introduction to the Data Retrieval Facilities of the XQt Language for Scientific Data

Javad Chamanara and Birgitta König-Ries

Friedrich-Schiller-University Jena, Heinz Nixdorf Endowed Chair for Distributed Information Systems, Ernst-Abbe-Platz 2, 07743 Jena, Germany
{javad.chamanara,birgitta.koenig-ries}@uni-jena.de
http://fusion.cs.uni-jena.de/

Abstract. Scientific data is stored in a wide variety of different formats. While much recent research and development have focused on specialized languages and tools to fulfill the requirements of specific domains or data structures, the need for more general technologies to enable data scientists to deal with various forms of data in a universal manner is growing. In this paper we describe data querying capabilities of the XQt language in order to show how it enables the users to author their processes in data source and format ignorant ways and to share and reuse their data, processes, and acquired skills. In addition, we describe the internals of the language, the execution pipeline, and the mapping between the domain level schemas and the physical structure of the data. The paper highlights the retrieval capabilities of XQt and illustrates some of its basic performance indicators.

1   Introduction

Data scientists deal with processing big, exploratory, and heterogeneous data. Usually they need to use several different tools to achieve their aim. Often these tools are not interoperable. Thus, it requires considerable effort to chain them into analysis pipelines [13]. Re-executing, documenting, or evaluating of these pipelines is also labor intensive. All these problems are particularly pronounced for scientific data as data integration from changing, heterogeneous sources across organizational boundaries plays such a big role.

A language that eases these processes would be of great value to data scientists. If the language supported sharing and reusing of data and process independently, this would be considerable add to this value.

In [4] we introduced the XQt[1] language and its runtime system – it aims at achieving these goals. A brief introduction to the language including its requirements, blueprint design and main elements is recaptured in Section 2. XQt aims at a full

---

[1] The language name has been changed to XQt (pronounced as execute) due to a name conflict with the work introduced in [11].

H. Galhardas and E. Rahm (Eds.): DILS 2014, LNBI 8574, pp. 143–150, 2014.

featured data querying and manipulation language, but in this paper, building on our previous work, we focus on its data retrieval facilities and defer the discussion of data manipulation and technical implementations to future work (Section 6).

XQt is a declarative, domain level, universal query language mainly designed to work with scientific data. Its declarative nature implies no ordering, no control statements, and immutable variables (Section 2). In order to work at the domain level, the language introduces the concept of "perspective", which allows scientists to author the specification of their data objects independent of the physical data structures stored in data sources. Processes authored in XQt are translated into the native language of the underlying data source with the help of dynamically chosen and loaded adapters (Section 3). For a data scientist it means that XQt offers a uniform way to query and process data regardless of the underlying data source. In addition, the XQt API allows other data processing software applications, i.e., Kepler [20], R [5], and Taverna [19] to hand over their data querying and management to XQt. The main features of some well-known data querying languages and systems that we modeled XQt upon are studied in related work (Section 5). Before summarizing the paper in Section 6, we present a preliminary performance evaluation of a CSV adapter prototype in Section 4.

2   XQt Design

XQt's design promotes a uniform data access mechanism through the development of a declarative language and its runtime system (See Fig. 2). We provide the needed expressive power while ensuring translatability to other languages or systems summarized in Section 5. Data querying facilities of XQt support the following elements.

1. Result Set Schema: defines the structure of the objects returned by the query in order to form a conceptual schema. Once the schema has been defined, it can be reused in all kinds of queries and for different underlying data sources.
2. Source Selection: specifies the data source the data should be retrieved from. It can be a single or joined data container or a previously populated variable.
3. Target Selection: Nominates an immutable variable to hold the result set of the query, to make it available for the following queries, functions, and visualizations.
4. Slicing: Skips over a number of objects in the result set and takes a specific number afterward.
5. Filtering: Removes the non-matching objects from the result set.
6. Ordering: Sorts the result set based on the provided sorting keys and directions.
7. Grouping: Groups the result set based on the grouping keys and/ or aggregation functions.
8. Anchoring: In hierarchical and graph data, the anchor defines the starting and/ or finishing patterns, so that the query operates in the defined scope.
9. Functions: A set of extendible functions available in filtering, grouping, and projection.

In XQt the term *process script,* or *process* for short, refers to a sequence of declarations and statements written in a specified order to serve as data processing requirements of a designated procedure. The *statement* is a unit of execution which may have a persistent effect on data. A *query* is a data retrieval statement without having any persistent (or side) effect on data. A *declaration* is a non-executable contract or a set of configuration items.

In the current XQt grammar one query syntax and three types of declarations are considered. Among the declarations, a *perspective* forms the data object schema from the domain point of view. A *connection* models the required information to get access to the data, and a *binding* establishes a relationship between a connection and a proper version of the data if a versioning scheme is in place. In addition, the binding scopes the set of underlying data containers visible to the statements. A query retrieves the data using the associated bindings and perspectives.

A perspective consists of a set of *attributes* defined locally, inherited from another perspective, or overridden the inherited ones. Each attribute describes one domain specific dimension of the data. The attribute's optional forward (read) and reverse (write) mappings are expressions able to perform data transformations such as type, format, and unit of measurement conversion, and data de/composition for retrieval and manipulation operations, respectively.

Fig. 1[2] illustrates the grammar of the query statement. The minimum query is constructed by a "SELECT" keyword followed by a source clause. The source selection clause specifies on which data the query should be executed. It can be a single or joined data container according to binding reference(s) or a previously defined variable. Target selection clause introduces a variable to keep the query result.

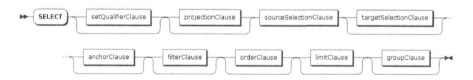

Fig. 1. The syntax diagram of SELECT statement

The projection clause explicitly nominates one of the previously declared perspectives as the query's result set schema. If not introduced, the query tries to infer it from the variable or binding scope(s) used as source. Filtering predicates are arithmetic and/ or logical expressions referring to the attributes of the bound perspective and previously defined variables. The result set can be ordered and/ or grouped using ordering and grouping clauses, respectively. The anchor clause expressions allow starting from and/ or stopping in a set of data objects. The limit clause trims the result set by taking a subset after optionally skipping a specific number of items. A simple query example is provided as part of the evaluation in Section 4.

---

[2] For space reasons, we left the description of "CONNECTION" and "BIND" out.

3   Query Execution

Execution of the statements begins with parsing of the input process, which includes syntax tree generation, statement completion and validation, and inter-element dependency control. When the process is successfully parsed, an annotator creates a Described Syntax Tree (DST), which contains a descriptor node for each element of the process, as well as for some of the remarkable phrases, e.g., expressions and variables. Indeed, the DST is the strongly typed and fully linked representation of the process. It acts as the intermediate grammar and data ignorant contract between the language and the adapters and API clients.

When the DST is ready, the query execution engine (QEE) executes all the statements. For each, using the binding information, the QEE chooses a proper registered adapter, passes the statement descriptor to it, and asks for execution. Upon receiving, the adapter transforms the descriptor from its domain level to a physical native counterpart if needed. The resulting native query is executed against the data. In cases the data source has no native query language or supporting runtime system, e.g., in CSV, and also if the chosen adapter does not provide all the capabilities asked for by the statement, a default adapter takes over partial responsibility of dealing with the data ensuring all the statements and their phrases are supported equally on all kinds of data sources. The QEE then assigns the result set to the nominated variable and keeps some internal tracks from the statement to the variable to the result set.

The final result set is held in an immutable ordered collection of data objects, each bound to the statement's perspective as the schema. The data types of perspective attributes are defined either explicitly or inferred from the mapping functions in accordance with the types of underlying fields. The language's type system is a subset of ISO: SQL 2008 types [8]. The language provides expressiveness components such as grouping, aggregation, and arithmetic operations [9, 10] as well as patterns, negation and expressions [1, 7], but does not support nesting and sub-queries.

4   Evaluation

We conducted a preliminary evaluation of the language to verify whether the language and its default CSV adapter are able to show an acceptable and linear performance over different sizes of data. To achieve this, we compared XQt's runtime for a set of typical sample queries to that of Postgres. Our aim was to see whether XQt's runtime performance is comparable to that of Postgres. The test was done using a 600 Megabytes CSV file of a slightly changed biodiversity dataset containing 10 million rows. Each row consists of timestamp, longitude (Degree), latitude (Degree), elevation (Meter), temperature (Celsius), and amount of soil nitrogen (microgram per volume unit) fields. We wanted the result set to include only rows having elevation between E1 and E2 Feet and temperature between T1 and T2 degree Fahrenheit, in that E1, E2, T1, and T2 can vary. Also in the result set, the elevation should be in Foot, the temperature in Fahrenheit and the soil nitrogen in Milligram per volume unit.

```
PERSPECTIVE soil
{
    ATTRIBUTE Timestamp: DateTime MapTo=timestamp,
    ATTRIBUTE Longitude: Real MapTo=longitude,
    ATTRIBUTE Latitude: Real MapTo=latitude,
    ATTRIBUTE Elevation: Real MapTo=elevation/0.3048,
    ATTRIBUTE Temperature: Real MapTo=1.8*temp+32,
    ATTRIBUTE SN: Double MapTo = soilNi / 1000,
}
CONNECTION cnn1 ADAPTER=CSV SOURCE_URI= "d:\data\"
PARAMETERS file_extension: csv
BIND b1 CONNECTION = cnn1  SCOPE = soildata1
SELECT PERSPECTIVE soil FROM b1.0 WHERE (Elevation>=0 AND
Elevation <=10 AND Temperature>=32 Temperature<=50)INTO
var1
```

Fig. 2. The process script that fetches and transforms data from a soil nitrogen observation dataset. It extracts the amount of soil nitrogen at different elevation/ temperatures. The adapter compiles the complete file name from the source_uri, scope and the file extension parameter. Binding b1.0 refers to the first scope, soildata1, defined in the b1 binding.

We ran the process depicted in Fig. 2 in XQt and its equivalent SELECT statement in Postgres having E1, E2, T1, and T2 parameters set to different values shown in Table 1 and measured the queries' execution time using the Java's built-in timer. Postgres data was loaded into a single table and indexed on the elevation and temperature fields before the test, but no special performance tuning was conducted.

Table 1. Performance of the XQt SELECT statement on a CSV dataset. The test has been done using the following configuration: CSV file size: 602 Megabytes, No. records: 10 Million, Operating System: Windows 7 Professional SP1, CPU: Intel Core i5/ M560/ 2.67 GHz/ 64 bits, Total Physical Memory: 8 GB, JVM: Java HotSpot^{TM} 64-Bit Server VM version 25.0-b67 (Java 8 beta), JVM Max Heap Size: 4 GB. Postgres version: 9.3.2. Both the XQt and Postgres APIs are called from the same application. XQt returns a java collection and Postgres a java ResultSet.

E1-E2 (M)	T1-T2 (F)	No. of Returned Records	PgS Time (Sec)	XQt Time (Sec)
00-00	32-32	0	4.93	7.89
290-323	32-47	107029	4.56	8.24
107-323	49-80	4061734	84.70	29.58
00-323	32-98	8054593	173.42	79.68
00-1200	32-122	10000000	216.60	95.24

The results of the test execution on XQt and Postgres are shown in Table 1. The XQt execution times show a linear response time. The difference between the first and last rows is almost consumed by performing object materialization, as Postgres executes the WHERE clause before the projection and XQt uses a two phase materialization.

5   Related Work

In order for XQt to be attractive to scientists, we need to make sure that a user can express virtually anything with XQt that she is used to being able to express with the query languages she used previously. Thus, a thorough look at a wide range of existing query languages was necessary. We studied query languages that are quite general in their respective data domains, e.g., relational, array based, XML, and graph data.

The Structured Query Language, SQL, is a relational data management language [10], operating on tables and queries [8]. The SELECT statement specifies the result set. The designated SQL-implementation translates the query into a query plan and executes it. The statement is comprised of smaller phrases; an optional set quantifier to determine whether the result set eliminates duplicates, a list of columns to appear in the result set, the table reference(s) from which data is to be retrieved, a search condition to eliminate all non-matching records from the result set, a grouping clause to put the records having common values together, a filtering conditions on the groups, a WINDOW clause to partition the result set, and apply aggregate functions to each partition and specify their ordering. A BNF representation of SQL grammar is available in [12].

SciDB is a multidimensional array DBMS [16] that uses Array Query Language (AQL), an SQL-like declarative language, for working with arrays. Queries written in AQL get compiled into Array Functional Language (AFL) and then passed through the processing pipeline [16]. An AQL query consists of projection, target, source, and filter elements. The AQL expressions can access the attributes and dimensions of the array as well as calling built-in functions. It is possible to join two or more arrays and use the joined array as the source of the query. Nested sub queries and aggregate functions are also supported.

A FLWOR, XQuery's expression language, statement is made up of FOR, LET, WHERE, ORDER BY, and RETURN clauses [2]. The FOR clause binds one or more iterator variables to input sequences. The LET clause assigns a value to a given immutable variable for a specific iteration. The optional WHERE clause filters the iteration in order to eliminate matching tuples generated by FOR and/ or LET clauses. The optional ORDER BY clause then imposes an order on the remaining tuples. The RETURN clause is executed for each tuple resulted from the previous clause, generating an ordered list of, possibly formatted, outputs. There is no grouping or distinction functionality in the expressions.

SPARQL [6] is a set of specifications that provide languages and protocols to query and manipulate RDF [3] data. It contains capabilities for querying required and optional graph patterns along with their conjunctions and disjunctions [7]. It also supports aggregation, sub queries, negation, and creating values by the use of expressions. Complex queries may include union, optional query parts, and filters.

The select query in SPARQL comprises of a SELECT clause, any number of DATASET clauses, a WHERE clause, and finally a solution modifier clause. The query executes on a set of RDF datasets [7] returning a solution set that matches imposed where clause conditions. It also supports function calls, union, offset and limit of the solution set.

Cypher is a declarative graph query language that allows querying and updating Neo4J graphs. According to its documentations described in [17], the query statement is close to the following description:

In Cypher, any query is describing a pattern in a graph. Patterns are expressions that return a collection of paths and are able to be evaluated as predicates. The MATCH clause allows specifying a search pattern used to match in the graph. The patterns can be introduced to match all nodes, nodes with a label, nodes having bidirectional or directed relationships, specific relationship types, calling functions that return patterns, and variable length relationship paths. The WITH clause divides a query into multiple, distinct parts, chaining subsequent query parts and forwards the results from one to the next [14]. Apart the MATCH clause, it is also possible to filter the result set using the WHERE clause. The query ends in a lazy RETURN clause which signals the end of the query. SKIP, LIMIT, and ORDER BY clauses are available after the RETURN clause.

BigSQL is the IBM's approach to deal with big data. It enables users to query data managed by Hadoop using an SQL like syntax by translating the SQL query to its Map-Reduce counterpart. BigSQL allows the user to import data from various sources into its tables in order to make them query-able. The tables' fields can be of complex or array types. It has a limited support for insert and no support for delete and update statements [15].

6   Conclusion and Future Work

In this paper we introduced the specification of the query statement of the XQt language and described how the runtime system accepts and executes the queries. Separation of schema definitions, connections, bindings, and statements increases process cleanness, and maintainability as well as enhancing sharing and skill transfer among users and tools. Perspectives provide a physical data ignorant mechanism by defining a domain level schema. The statements can be executed against different versions of the same data, in different formats, or in different storages by applying minimal changes in the process script. Having various viewpoints on the same data, e.g., for different processing or visualization purposes, is as easy as defining multiple perspectives. The language is implemented using EBNF[3] in ANTLR 4[4]. The runtime system is under active development and we are testing its integration with a CSV adapter developed for this purpose. The future work on the language adds adapters for other commonly used data sources as well as providing join, versioning support, and data manipulation functionalities. The language will be integrated into BExIS [18] and thoroughly evaluated in the context of biodiversity data.

---

[3] Extended Backus–Naur Form,
 https://en.wikipedia.org/wiki/Extended_Backus-Naur_Form
[4] ANTLR Version 4, http://www.antlr.org/

Acknowledgements. The work described in this article is done in the context of BExIS++ [18] project. BExIS++ is funded by DFG (German Research Foundation) within the LIS program.

References

1. Angles, R., Gutierrez, C.: The Expressive Power of SPARQL. In: Sheth, A.P., Staab, S., Dean, M., Paolucci, M., Maynard, D., Finin, T., Thirunarayan, K. (eds.) ISWC 2008. LNCS, vol. 5318, pp. 114–129. Springer, Heidelberg (2008)
2. Boag, S., Chamberlin, D.D., Fernández, M.F., Florescu, D., Robie, J., Siméon, J.: XQuery 1.0: An XML Query Language, 2nd edn. (2010)
3. Carroll, J., Klyne, G.: Resource Description Framework (RDF): Concepts and Abstract Syntax. W3C (2004)
4. Chamanara, J., König-Ries, B.: SciQL: a query language for unified scientific data processing and management. PIKM, 17–24 (2012)
5. Gentleman, R., Ihaka, R.: R Statistical Language (2012), http://www.r-project.org
6. W3C SPARQL Working Group: SPARQL 1.1 Overview, Recommendation REC-sparql11-overview-20130321 (2013)
7. Harris, S., Seaborne, A.: SPARQL 1.1 Query Language. W3C (2013)
8. ISO 2008. Information Technology, Database Languages, SQL, Part 1: Framework, SQL/Framework (2008)
9. ISO 1992. ISO/ IEC 9075:1992: Title: Information technology — Database languages — SQL. International Organization for Standardization (1992)
10. ISO 1999. ISO/ IEC 9075-2:1999: Information technology — Database languages — SQL — Part 2: Foundation, SQL/ Foundation (1999)
11. Kersten, M., Zhang, Y., Ivanova, M., Nes, N.: a query language for science applications. In: Proceedings of the EDBT/ICDT 2011 Workshop on Array Databases, Uppsala, Sweden, pp. 1–12 (2011)
12. Leffler, J.: BNF Grammar for ISO/IEC 9075-2:2003, SQL/Foundation (2012)
13. Prabhu, P., Jablin, T.B., Raman, A., Zhang, Y., Huang, J., Kim, H., Johnson, N.P., Liu, F., Ghosh, S., Beard, S., Oh, T., Zoufaly, M., Walker, D., August, D.I.: A Survey of the Practice of Computational Science. In: SC 2011 State of the Practice Reports, pp. 1–12 (2011)
14. Robinson, I., Webber, J., Eifrem, E.: Graph Databases. O'Reilly Media (2013)
15. Saracco, C.M., Jain, U.: What's the big deal about Big SQL (2013), http://www.ibm.com/developerworks/library/bd-bigsql/ (visited April 2014)
16. Stonebraker, M., Brown, P., Poliakov, A., Raman, S.: The architecture of sciDB. In: Bayard Cushing, J., French, J., Bowers, S. (eds.) SSDBM 2011. LNCS, vol. 6809, pp. 1–16. Springer, Heidelberg (2011)
17. The Neo4J Team, The Neo4J Manual. Neo Technology (2013)
18. BExIS++ (Biodiversity Exploratory Information System), http://fusion.cs.uni-jena.de/bexis (visited April 2014)
19. Taverna Workflow Management System, http://www.taverna.org.uk (visited December 2013)
20. The Kepler Project, https://kepler-project.org (visited December 2013)

Author Index